Tennis Elbow Relief

Serving up solutions for lateral epicondylitis

Tennis Elbow Relief
Published by: Emma Green Programs
61 S Baldwin Avenue #712
Sierra Madre CA 91024
USA
Contact publisher for permission requests.

The information provided in this book is designed to provide helpful information on the subjects discussed. This book is not meant to be used, nor should it be used, to diagnose or treat any medical condition. For diagnosis or treatment of any medical problem, consult your own physician.

ISBN: 978-1-7368460-0-1

Cover design by Leesa Ellis
Interior book design & formatting by Leesa Ellis
Photography by Beth Moser

$1 from the sale of this book goes to support the amazing work of Dachshunds and Friends Rescue. "A home for every dog and a dog for every home."

Emma Green
The Tennis Elbow Queen

presents

Tennis Elbow Relief

Serving up solutions for lateral epicondylitis

**Learn the fundamental steps
that take you from hurt to healed!**

Essential reading for people who are ready
to resolve elbow pain for good.

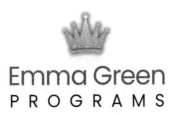

Emma Green
P R O G R A M S

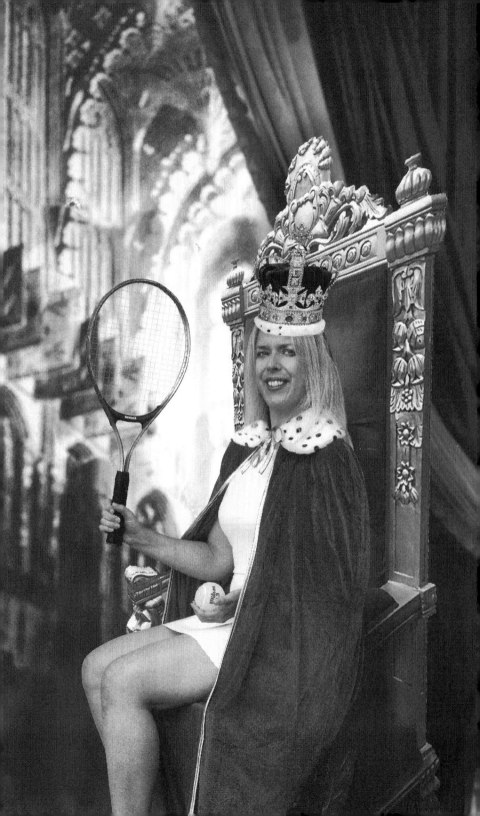

This book is dedicated to my family
and my clients.

My family for supporting me through
everything I want to achieve.

My clients, without whom,
this book wouldn't exist.

You are the reason I do what I do.
You are the reason I work every day.
To see you recover from debilitating injuries,
witnessing your transformations, and regaining
the lives you want to live is a gift.
I am truly humbled to share this journey
with you and honored that you entrust me
with your care.

TENNIS ELBOW QUEEN Contents

Welcome i

Foreword by Buddy Gibbons iii

Introduction vii

Who Is This Book For? ix

Chapter 1 Could Everything You've Been Told
About Tennis Elbow Be Wrong? 1

   1. You must play tennis to get tennis elbow. 4

   2. Rest it and it will go away by itself, eventually. 5

   3. An injection will cure it. 7

   4. Surgery is the only option. 10

   5. Once you've got it, you've got it for life,
there's nothing you can do. You'll just have
to live with it and take pain pills. 11

   6. You only get it in your dominant arm,
but then it will spread to the other arm. 13

   7. Anti-inflammatory medication will help
as my elbow has been inflamed for months. 15

   8. It's my age and my parents had it,
so I guess it's going to be the same for me. 17

   9. I need an x-ray or an MRI scan
to see what's wrong. 20

   10. Exercise will make it worse and I'm in
too much pain to come to therapy. 21

   11. "I had physical therapy, and it didn't work." 22

   COVID-19 Update 25

Chapter 2 The Most Common Mistakes You Can Make
If You Have Tennis Elbow 29

   Doing Nothing 29

   Pain Pills 30

   Injections 31

   Surgery 32

Brace / Strap / Clasp 35

Rest 36

Exercises From YouTube 37

Massage 38

Ultrasound And Other Electrotherapy 39

Chapter 3   Why Did You Get Tennis Elbow? 41

Overuse 41

Altered Biomechanics 44

Direct Trauma 44

Compensation Mechanism 45

Antibiotics 45

Ergonomics 45

Chapter 4   What's Tennis Elbow? 49

Why It Can Last So Long 54

What Is Pain? 55

Chronic Pain 55

Why Do Anything About A Bit Of A Niggle? 57

Chapter 5   Why Do You Need A Guide? 61

Phase 1 61

Phase 2 62

Phase 3 62

Phase 4 63

Which Phase Are You In? 63

Chapter 6   Phase 1: Self-Help Strategies 69

The Power Of The Right Solution 69

Heat The Heck Out Of It 69

Ice, Ice, Baby 71

Posture Rules 73

Relative Rest 79

Ergonomics 80

Braces 81

Sleep 82

Pills, Potions And Lotions 84

Nutrition...85

Hydration...87

Cardio Exercise 87

Mental Cardio..90

Relaxation..91

Meditation 94

Visualization 96

Quick Recap...99

Chapter 7   Phase 2: Normalizing The Soft Tissues.............. 103

Getting Soft For The Soft Tissues 103

We Should Learn From The Animals....................104

Joints Are Designed To Move...............................106

The Best 3 Stretches That We All Should
Be Doing...107

    Knee Rolling..107

    Neck Retractions (a.k.a. Chin Tucks).................109

    Upper Traps Stretch 109

Self-Massage...111

Chapter 8   Phase 3: Strengthening 113

Breathing 114

Core Of Steel.. 114

Why Your Core Lets You Down
When You Need It Most.......................................119

How Do You Strengthen Your Core?....................120

The Best Core Exercise... Ever 121

Why This Is Crucial For Your Recovery 124

Chapter 9   Phase 4: Endurance And Function.................... 127

How Long Does Each Phase Take? 128

Nerve Mobilisations 130

Chapter 10   Next Steps 133

30-Day And 100-Day Guides.................................133

Facebook Group...133

Helpful Hints Emails..134

Tennis Elbow Relief Challenge 134

Website 135

Tennis Elbow Relief Program 135

Membership Group 136

Your Opportunity To Work With Emma
Beyond This Book 136

Telehealth 138

Success Stories 141

Your 30-Day Starting Boost Plan 147

(Phase 1 And The Beginning Of
Phases 2 And 3) 148

Before You Start 148

The Basic Guidelines 148

Worksheets 149

The Next 100 Days Program 157

(Phase 3 And Phase 4) 157

Bonus Section 161

Boost Your Immunity
And Emma's Extra Energy 161

Daily Exercise 162

Getting Into Nature 162

Daily Meditation 162

Daily Journaling 163

Daily Multivitamins 163

Better Nutrition 163

Quarantini Time 164

Gratitude 165

FAQs 167

How does your Program help tennis elbow? 167

What makes your Program different to other
treatments out there? 167

Questions to ask your healthcare provider 167

Do you suggest doing stretches in the morning
even when you don't have any pain? 168

Should we stretch before or after exercise? 168

Does my insurance cover me coming to see you? ..169

I can get Physical Therapy much more cheaply.
What makes you different? 171

Can Foam Rolling help? 172

Does Kinesio Tape work for tennis elbow? 172

What is the recommended usage? 173

Should I do yoga? 174

References 175

Acknowledgments 181

About The Author 183

Welcome

Welcome to a growing group of people who are taking their health into their own hands and healing themselves. They may have tried many other solutions in the past, but nothing seemed to help. So, they took responsibility for their own health and searched out a better way to heal themselves.

Within the pages of this book, you will find many strategies to heal lateral epicondylitis, aka tennis elbow. Some you most likely have tried before. Some will be new to you. Trust the process. This program has worked for thousands of elbows all over the world and now is in a format to help you. I wanted to write a book that someone could pick up and heal their tennis elbow themselves. Is every single one of my strategies and techniques in here? No, they're not. That would have become overwhelming and you wouldn't make it all the way through.

There are over 10 bonus checklists, calendars, videos and worksheets in downloadable form. To get full access to the bonus section (all the extra resources I mention in this book, and other goodies I couldn't fit in here), make sure you sign up for free at:

http://bit.ly/TE-bookbonuses

Although we are not directly working together, I'm here with you on this journey. I've included links to my website, videos, worksheets and groups to aid you in your journey to healing. Don't hesitate to reach out if you have any questions. I LOVE questions!

So, without further ado, let's hear from someone who was instrumental in the formation of this program. But for them, this book wouldn't be in your hands right now!

Foreword

BY BUDDY GIBBONS

I am a professional drummer. You've heard me play on thousands of television commercials, broadcasts, sports shows, and film scores. You've never heard OF me, but you've heard me.

But that almost wasn't my life at all.

The year was 2008. My wife and I had moved to Los Angeles after a stint in Nashville. I knew that I had to work incredibly hard to establish myself in the uber-competitive LA music scene. I searched out work in every nook and cranny of the Craigslist, the LA Weekly, The Recycler, and I took every gig that I could... over 300 of them. I began having some trouble with my right arm... numbness, tingling, pain. Eventually, the pain became so intense that I could no longer lift a bottle of water. I had to hug a pillow any time I was sitting, just so that I could keep my arm in a specific position where it didn't hurt quite as badly. As you can imagine, that made things quite difficult for someone in my line of work. I had played my arm to death. It was time to seek medical help.

I began with my general practitioner. She couldn't figure out what the problem was, because my symptoms didn't perfectly match any of the syndromes/problems/injuries she was familiar with. So, we decided to go the route of cortisone shots. Over the next year and a half, I had so many shots that I actually considered getting an "X" tattooed on the spot where my elbow pain originated. I figured I could take out the guesswork that way. But the reality was that the shots weren't a cure, they were only a treatment, and my career was in serious jeopardy. I sought out a surgeon and ran across some seriously questionable ideas about fixing my elbow, not the least of which was the suggestion by a doctor who wanted to take a hammer and chisel to my bones, only to give me a 70% chance of recovery. No thanks! Finally, I met a truly caring surgeon in Pasadena, and she said to me, "I can't fix your elbow, but I have an idea..." That idea was to get me into Occupational Therapy.

My Occupational Therapist was a wonderful person, and I could tell that she was both sympathetic and empathetic to my situation. We worked for several months, with little to no change in my pain level and functionality. My body had begun to shut down in other ways as well. Muscles were tightening all over my body. I was no longer moving in a normal manner at all. Photos taken of me during that time show that I was wearing 'pain face' everywhere I went. I still have a hard time looking at pictures from that time in my life. In the meantime, my case became something of a talking point in the hospital's therapy department. It was finally determined that the best chance I had for recovery was to move from occupational therapy to physical therapy.

Enter, Emma Green.

Long before she was 'The Tennis Elbow Queen', she was just the latest person in whom I was putting my hope. My previous experience with Physical Therapy had not been particularly positive, but I was desperate for help. She walked into the room, this tiny English lady, with a charming smile and a deeply caring demeanor. I could feel how much interest she had in me and my case. Beyond her obvious 'care', however, was a keenly curious mind. She wanted to figure me out. She wanted to help me. We began my therapy sessions... they did not go well. I was getting quite frustrated because for the first few weeks, we never touched my elbow. Finally, in my despair, I asked her to PLEASE explain to me why we were working on my back... my shoulder... my big toe (not really)! So, she calmly took me down the hall to meet "Henry", the life-sized, half muscle, half bone skeleton in the other exam room. She showed me how my muscles, tendons, ligaments, and bones connected to each other, and how one movement was part of the bigger picture of many movements. My neck and back were so tight that there was no way my elbow would be able to heal until she got the rest of my body moving the correct way. From that moment on, I knew that, no matter how long it took, I was going to be ok. She really did understand. She saw the big picture.

A few weeks went by and I achieved a modicum of progress on my neck and shoulders. In fact, I could now turn my head like a normal person! Then it happened: "Buddy, I've got an idea". I was certain I'd heard that line before. So what, exactly, was Emma's idea? She had devised a therapy for the elbow based on the science of repairing an Achilles tendon. She explained in great detail how she could see the principles of the Achilles treatment working to repair the damage inside my elbow.

So, we began. Day one, she showed me the exercise. I was skeptical. After all, what good would an exercise with a 1lb weight do me, a 6'2", 230lb, athletically built man? I scoffed at the idea... until I couldn't complete the movement with that small amount of weight. That's how damaged my elbow was. That's how much pain I was in. She instructed me to go home and do that exercise twice a day, three sets. It was difficult to admit just how weak I was. It was embarrassing. It was frustrating, but I did the work. Eventually, I could get through the sets with one pound. Then two pounds. I began to feel a little bit of relief. I didn't hurt constantly. I didn't have to sleep with a pillow tucked into my arm every single night. Each visit with Emma, she'd measure my grip strength and put me through the paces of the exercise. She'd still mobilize my back and shoulders, she'd push me to increase the weight.

Then came 'that' Tuesday morning. I'll never forget it. I'd gotten up and was fixing myself a bowl of Cap'n Crunch. I reached into the refrigerator, took out the milk, poured it over the cereal, replaced the milk in the fridge, and closed the door... with my damaged right arm! I had no pain at all. In fact, it felt so natural that I didn't realize what I'd done until I was half way into the living room with my prized sugary treat! When it hit me, I sat the bowl down, again with my right arm, and began to sob. I called my wife and told her what had happened. She cried at her office. We celebrated that night as if it was the biggest news we'd ever gotten. Why?

Because that was the moment I got my life back.

It's been over a decade now, and my elbow is still as good as new. If I ever feel any issues coming on, I turn to the exercises Emma created for me and I'm back to 100% within a day or two. The gratitude and love I feel for Emma is many levels deep. I'm thrilled that the techniques she created for my issues have helped so many other people overcome their own elbow problems. It wasn't always easy, but it was miraculous for me.

I'll always be indebted to, and thankful for, the tiny English woman who healed my elbow. My friend, "The Tennis Elbow Queen", Emma Green.

– Buddy Gibbons
Drummer • Composer • Producer

Introduction

Hello. I am Emma Green and I'm the Tennis Elbow Queen! I'm actually a physical therapist, or physiotherapist as we are known in some parts of the world. I was born, raised and trained in the UK, working there for a little over 10 years before relocating to the USA, and jumping through all of the red tape to get my physical therapy license in California. That was 15 years ago now. So, I've been a PT for a very long time. Probably longer than some of you have been alive!

In my previous life, when I was working in the UK, I worked with a number of different sports teams. I got to travel all over the world, to many different countries, helping athletes compete at the very highest level. Then, when I moved to the USA and had a couple of kids, the traveling slowed down. My practice changed from working with professional athletes to working with professional musicians. They didn't need me to travel with them, but their mindset, drive and work ethic was no different to the athletes I was so used to helping.

What was different though was the type of injuries that I was seeing. The athletes I commonly worked with would injure their backs, knees and ankles, while the musicians would complain about their necks, shoulders and elbows.

After an incredibly comprehensive education working at a large regional teaching hospital in the National Health Service in the UK, I had spent 6 months working alongside a Shoulder

Consultant and 6 months working in a hand unit. This gave me great insight into the musicians' movement patterns and mechanisms of injury.

This new direction began when I was asked by a co-worker of mine, who is a Certified Hand Therapist, to assess a professional drummer she was treating for Tennis Elbow. The drummer, Buddy (he tells his story in the foreword to this book), was desperate for answers to his problem as he couldn't play and so couldn't make a living and anyone who knows a musician knows that making music is not just what they do, but it's who they are. Buddy had had that taken away from him.

He was truly miserable, and borderline depressed. He and his wife had traveled the country looking for a solution to his Tennis Elbow and had so far failed. Acupuncture, chiropractic treatment, massage, stretches, doctors, cortisone shots...nothing worked. He ended up in a surgeon's office begging for surgery to alleviate his pain. Thankfully, she refused until he had seen one of her trusted therapists; that is, the Certified Hand Therapist I shared an office with at the time.

After I evaluated Buddy, it became patently clear that there was way more going on than "**Just** a Tennis Elbow." How many times have you heard that phrase from people who have clearly never suffered with Tennis Elbow? During the time I worked with Buddy, I trawled the research to come up with the very best, latest and evidence-based treatments for tendon healing that I could find. There was nothing there for Tennis Elbow. The research was very good at telling us what didn't work, but not as good at telling us what did. So, I devised a brand-new program, something that had never seen before, to treat Buddy and get him back to doing what he loves, playing the drums.

After he healed, he went back to the surgeon's office for a

check-up appointment. She called me soon after and asked me what new treatments I was doing that had been so effective for someone who had been told there was a strong chance he would never likely be able to play the drums again. I shared with her my program and a strong working relationship was born. She still sends me all her Tennis Elbow clients to this day 13 years after I first worked with Buddy. I'm proud to call her a friend.

Let me share my program with you. Read on my friend, read on.

Who Is This Book For?

Research shows that about 2% of the adult population will have Tennis Elbow at some point in their lives [1.] This is the reason, I think, that there is so little research done on this problem and so few truly effective treatments.

My first recollection of the term "Tennis Elbow" came as a child. My Mum was diagnosed with Lateral Epicondylitis, aka Tennis Elbow, probably due to looking after 3 kids and keeping house, and the treatment she was given was a cortisone injection, nothing else, no therapy, no exercises, just straight in with a shot. I can remember her saying it was the most painful thing she had ever endured, and she'd had 3 children. Sadly, her pain came back and she underwent another injection. Boy, Tennis Elbow must have been pretty bad if you were going to go through 2 intensely painful injections to try to get rid of it.

I guess that's why I subconsciously did everything in my power to help Buddy heal. When I met him, I was in a position to utilize my skills to solve his problem, something that my Mum had been unable to find years before. That's how my Tennis Elbow Relief program came into being. It's been refined over the years as new research has come out, and it's evolved to be effective as a remote treatment option. It's helped clients all over the world.

This book is for those people who have searched for solutions to their Tennis Elbow pain but have been failed. There's a ton of information out there regarding this subject and, unfortunately, not all of it is correct. Here I take you through the whats, whys and wherefores of working towards resolving your own Tennis Elbow.

Let me help you heal. Read on.

CHAPTER 1

Could Everything You've Been Told About Tennis Elbow Be Wrong?

The short answer would be... yes. However, to explain a little further and start to understand why some of these legends have evolved, I've picked out a few of the most commonly heard myths surrounding Tennis Elbow.

There's a lot of misinformation out there regarding lateral epicondylitis or Tennis Elbow and I guess it's because so many of us have either suffered from it at some point or another, or know someone who has. Indeed, the US Department of Health and Human Services, National Institutes of Health, cite 2% of people will suffer from Tennis Elbow pain at some point in their lives [2]. I've been a Physical Therapist for a long time and guess this is about right. The average general physical therapist, who sees everything and everybody, backs, necks, knees, elbows, and so on, will see 1 or 2 Tennis Elbows per year, So, that statistic is likely accurate. My caseload is a little different with over 75% of my clients suffering with Tennis Elbows.

Just Google "Tennis Elbow Treatment" if you haven't already and count the list of suggestions you get. It's infinite.

How do you know what's right for you? Great question.

How do you know if something's wrong for you? Even better question.

So, you browse for a few minutes and then what? You do nothing. It's ok, we all do it. It's called Analysis Paralysis, too many options causing you to be overwhelmed, and so we don't do any of them. Best to keep yourself safe, eh? I'll just see how it goes... Wait... what, you think it's going to suddenly and miraculously get better, even though you've been suffering with it for weeks, months or even years?

You know, once you start telling people "I've got tennis elbow", or you start putting a strap on your arm and people see you've got tennis elbow, they're going to give you little bits of advice, all the things they've heard, all the old wives' tales, the myths. So, I have collated the top myths that clients of mine have told me over the past 13 years, and I'm going to go through each one and tell you why these are not true.

Here are the top things people have told me about having Tennis Elbow pain:

- You must play tennis to get tennis elbow.
- Rest it and it will go away by itself, eventually.
- An injection will cure it.
- Surgery is the only option.
- Once you've got it, you've got it for life, there's nothing you can do. You'll just have to live with it and take pain pills.
- You only get it in your dominant arm, but then it likely will spread to the other arm.

- Anti-inflammatory medication helps as that elbow has been inflamed for months.
- It's my age and my parents had it, so I guess it's going to be the same for me.
- I need an X-ray or an MRI scan to see what's wrong.
- Exercise will make it worse and I'm in too much pain to come to therapy (my all-time favorite).
- Physical Therapy didn't work for me. (Urgh, this is like a knife to my gut.)

Any of these sound familiar?

Let's take a deeper look at some of these myths.

You wake up one sunny morning and spring out of bed, ready to enjoy the day, when BAM. Suddenly, you are hit with the pain on the outside of your elbow. What is going on? Is it serious? What should you do? You cross to the bathroom and search around the medicine cabinet for some anti-inflammatory or pain pills. You hate taking pills, but this pain is so bad. But which pills should you take? You're not sure, So, you start trying to read the damn small writing on the side of the bottle, while the pain seems to be spreading down your arm. Then, you give in on trying to read the label and take two pain pills. That's got to be ok, right?

You look at your reflection in the mirror and don't recognize the face contorted with agony. As you look over your shoulder in the mirror, your gaze rests on the shower. A nice hot shower. That'll work, won't it? Wait, should you be using heat or ice? I don't know. Why oh, why is this so hard? So, you forgo the shower and head into the kitchen to make your coffee. As you do so, you reach out to pick up your favorite mug. YIIIIIIOOOOOWWWCCCHHH... That was not a good idea as the pain is now down to your wrist. Oh, when will the pain pills kick in?

This pain is so bad, there has to be something seriously wrong, right?

Recognize this kind of story? In this situation, the worst part is the not-knowing what to do for the best. I'm going to explain this scenario and more as you read through this book.

Let's investigate the following concerns that clients have shared with me;

1. You must play tennis to get tennis elbow.

This must be the number one thing people say regarding tennis elbow. "How can I have tennis elbow? I don't play tennis!" In fact, most people who are suffering with tennis elbow, have never picked up a racquet in their lives. Now, there's always an exception to the rule, and some do get tennis elbow from playing tennis.

Have you ever played tennis? Or are you a tennis player? I would say out of all the clients I've worked with, the thousands of elbows I've seen over the past 13 years, probably 5% are tennis players. Probably 8% play some kind of racket sport, maybe it's not tennis, maybe it's squash, or maybe it's pickleball. Tennis Elbow is the layman's term for the problem that you have with your elbow. The official medical diagnosis for Tennis Elbow is Lateral Epicondylitis.

A tennis coach once told me that he considers tennis elbow in tennis players, to be "Bad Stroke-itis", meaning that people who use poor form while playing tennis are the ones who go on to develop tennis elbow. This can be true, but it can also occur from simply overuse, even with a good technique. If someone jumped from playing tennis occasionally to suddenly playing for 3 hours every day, the tissues involved in gripping and swinging the racquet would complain about how much extra work they were having to do, while not being used to it. A little bit like we would ache like mad if we went and worked out hard at the gym if we weren't used to it. However, you do not have to play tennis to get tennis elbow.

The large majority of people suffering with tennis elbow develop it over time, from overuse through other activities, such as painting their house, using a screwdriver, playing a musical instrument, traveling, repetitive lifting at work or at home, housework, cleaning, renovating a property, increasing or changing their workout in the gym, repetitive movements at work, excessive computer use, keyboarding or mouse use, prolonged tablet or phone use...the list goes on and on.

The good news is that no matter how you developed tennis elbow, the same program will resolve it. Read on to find out more...

2. Rest it and it will go away by itself, eventually.

The second myth, "Rest will cure it."

Rest from any aggravating activities is an essential part of the healing of tennis elbow. However, rest by itself, will not cure tennis elbow and get the sufferer back doing all the activities they have been missing out on, with no restrictions. The reason being is that because most people suffer from tennis elbow for a long period of time, the muscles involved, which are attached to the painful tendon, become weak. Therefore, each time you use the muscle, the tendon gets pulled upon and that's irritating to the injured tendon. So, because it hurts, we do it less. If we do that activity less, the tendon doesn't get pulled on, but consequently, the attached muscle doesn't get used, leading to the muscle getting weaker and weaker the longer it's not used.

Continuing to stay away from any aggravating activity now gives the tendon a chance to start to settle down. Yay. We're heading in the right direction, but slow down because once you feel a bit better, you might start to think about picking up that tennis racquet, or whatever activity it happens to be. You get excited at the prospect of getting back to normal and returning to all the fun things you love to do and as soon as you try to lift the heavy saucepan, or whatever activity makes you happy, you feel that familiar pain and your arm feels incredibly weak. Because it is. You've rested from irritating activities for long enough so that the tendon has started to heal, but because the muscles haven't been doing anything and they are still super weak, the structure cannot tolerate the stresses and strains of normal daily activities that you are now starting to do. And guess what? Then the tendon starts to become irritated again... Vicious circle...

Rest will help. Absolutely it will, and I use relative rest as part of my program.

Relative rest is helpful when we're talking about tennis elbow, but total rest is not going to cure it. As we've just learned, total rest will actually weaken the muscles that support the elbow, causing more stress and strain to go through the injured area. It's a much better idea to gently keep moving and changing position as your body tells you. Our bodies are very perceptive, we should listen to them more often.

Rest will decrease your symptoms. I hear this so often from clients who say, "If I don't play tennis, work out, play my musical instruments, play with my kids, pick my kids up, lift the groceries, pick up a bottle of water... If I don't do those things, I'm fine." It doesn't sound like living to me. That's no fun. We will use rest, but it isn't going to cure the problem. There are other things that will cure it.

Tennis Elbow does not heal itself. Tendons are notoriously stubborn. You may have heard people talking about different issues and saying, "Oh, I used to have problems with my back and then I woke up one day and those problems had gone." This will not happen with a tennis elbow. The reason is that, due to the pathology of the tendon, the pain does not go away by itself, and we'll delve deeper into this later in the book. Your symptoms can settle down, they absolutely can, but you won't be back doing everything you want to do because that tendon has not healed. The pain will come back, and it always comes back if you don't heal it correctly and many times it will feel worse each time it recurs too.

3. An injection will cure it.

Not true. Recent research has shown that multiple injections of steroid (cortisone) into a soft tissue, can weaken the structure of the soft tissue and cause it to fail, not only leading to a prolonged healing time, but also poorer outcomes [3]. That's not good. So, if someone says to you, "Cortisone injections are the best treatment for tennis elbow", that is not true. If only it were that simple. If you've ever been prescribed oral steroids for an infection, you may have noticed, "Oh my goodness, I feel amazing. My joints don't ache and my back's ok." Steroids can do that and cortisone is a steroid. But, read on.

Back in the fifties, sports doctors found that if they injected steroids into the joints and soft tissues of football players who were injured, they could get them on the field every week, week in and week out. They could get these injured players out there and they were excited, "This is fantastic. All we've got to do is just hit them with an injection and out they go to play."

However, a few years later, what happened is that these

football players started to fall apart. Quite literally. What we know now is that if you have too many cortisone shots into one area in your lifetime, the steroid starts to degrade the soft tissues [4.] It starts to break down the soft tissues. That's not good. Some players would get tendon ruptures. The muscle tissue was breaking down and their ligaments would start to degrade. The sports doctors were not happy about this and they started looking into what was happening to the players. They realized that it was too much cortisone.

Fast forward to today and most doctors are decreasing the number of steroid shots they are performing for pathologies such as tennis elbow. The realization has become apparent that shots for tennis elbow don't get rid of the symptoms, they may just mask them for a few weeks before the original symptoms return with a vengeance. Add to this the possibility of side-effects that come with an invasive procedure like an injection, and it becomes clear why the administering of steroid injections for tennis elbow is not the optimum course of action.

I work very closely with a surgeon who's an upper limb specialist. She helps clients who have shoulder, elbow, wrist and hand problems. She does not do cortisone shots at all anymore into tennis elbows. She doesn't need to because she sends these clients to me. These patients don't need them. She describes it to them as a band aid for their symptoms.

It's a band aid, not a cure, and there are side effects [5, 6] such as;

- It can degrade the soft tissues including cartilage, tendon and skin as I mentioned with the football players and cause tendon ruptures.

- It's an invasive procedure. It's not a hugely invasive procedure, but there's still a needle going in, so it is possible to get an infection in that area.

- Discoloration, or a depigmentation of the skin around that area can occur. It is rare, but is a possibility.
- Fat atrophy can also happen. The steroid affects and reduces the subcutaneous fat just under the skin and it can make the elbow look a little unusual in that you start to really see the bony area. Normally we have muscle, we have fat, we have fascia, we have different soft tissues that make up our body and the cortisone can take away all of the fat from the surrounding area and it makes the little bump on the elbow look much more prominent.
- Steroid flare, this can include a temporary increase in pain at the site.
- Temporary facial flushing.
- Disturbed menstrual pattern.
- Skin rash, including cellulitis.
- Temporary blood sugar spike.
- Thinning or death of nearby bone (osteoporosis or osteomyelitis).
- Nerve damage.
- Increased risk of injury recurrence.

So, for many reasons, cortisone shots are not the best treatment. They're not a helpful option. Consequently, I am very conservative when it comes to invasive procedures such as these. My belief is that you should have no more than three cortisone injections into any one part of your body in your entire lifetime. Now, the good thing is that to successfully heal tennis elbow you don't need steroid injections at all. This is an outdated form of treatment. If anybody suggests an injection to you, run in the opposite direction. The fantastic news is that there are far more effective treatments that can completely resolve tennis elbow and not have it return and are non-invasive. I call that a win Win WIN.

4. Surgery is the only option.

Surgery of any kind should always be the absolute last resort. The reason is that, once a tissue has been cut, it will never be 100% again. It can't be. Soft tissues which are cut repair themselves with scar tissue, not the original tissue. That is, muscle tissue doesn't heal with muscle tissue, it heals with scar tissue. Ligaments don't heal with ligament tissue; they heal with scar tissue. Cut tendons don't heal with tendon tissue, they heal with scar tissue. You get the picture?

The reason this is so important to understand is that, once a tissue heals with scar tissue it is obviously not completely normal as there's an area of essentially abnormal tissue within its structure. This creates a potential weak spot. Guess where abnormal stress and strain are likely to show up again in the future? You got it. At those "weak" spots. So, ideally, surgery should be avoided unless it is absolutely the last resort.

There is good news though. The treatment protocol I teach reverses the degeneration of the tendon, which allows the tendon to heal without the addition of scar tissue. The way it does this is by the specific stress and strain loaded through the tendon. You'll learn how to do this safely later on in this book.

The surgeon I work with doesn't do tennis elbow surgeries anymore because she sends those clients to me. She is a surgeon who does surgery, but she will not do tennis elbow surgeries because oftentimes, they are not necessary. So, again, if somebody says, "Oh, we've done the shot and it didn't work. Let's try surgery", that probably isn't the best course of action. Once you start doing any kind of invasive procedures into that area, you start getting scar tissue building up. You can start impinging nerves within that scar tissue. Your elbow will never be the same again, ever. It just won't. It can't be because there's scar tissue in there that wasn't there before. If we heal it, non-surgically and non-invasively that elbow can be as good, if not actually, I think, better than it was before.

Every conservative form of treatment should be investigated before undergoing surgery, and that follows true for any issue. It's upsetting for people to believe that having surgery will cure them and when they wake up, they are still feeling symptoms. Surgery is not a panacea.

5. Once you've got it, you've got it for life, there's nothing you can do. You'll just have to live with it and take pain pills.

Let's just backtrack a little bit to number two; remember "Rest will cure it"? Well, rest can make it better, but it will always come back if it hasn't healed correctly. But does it always have to come back? No, if you heal it correctly, there is absolutely no reason why it should come back. That is what I'm going to teach you in this book; how to heal it correctly.

Do you want to keep managing episodic elbow pain over time because it will keep coming back or do you want to absolutely get rid of it once and for all? Most people say to me, "Yes, I want to get rid of it for good." That is the recognition of not just getting to the point of being pain-free, but additionally what else needs to be done to get to the point where the tendon is healed, and not going to come back again? Essentially, you can get yourself to the pain free point if you do not use your arm. You have rested the tendon and the symptoms have settled down. Great, you think to yourself, I am cured! But hold on, the tendon is still injured and will likely let you know as soon as you try to lift your cup of coffee with that arm again.

If you take an ultrasound scan of an affected tendon, many times the tendon looks thickened, compared to a normal tendon [7.] This is due to the pathology of tennis elbow. Resting it, or using basic therapies, can allow the irritated tendon to start to settle down. But even if a patient feels pain free, the ultrasound scan would reveal no change in the appearance of the tendon. It would still look exactly the same as it did at the height of the problem. Therefore, the symptoms can keep coming back because the underlying pathology has not changed, so, it's really easy for the symptoms to return. There are now treatments that reverse this pathology. Yes, the tendon returns to normal. Keep reading to find out more.

Regarding "There's nothing I can do to help it". There's always something you can do, but guidance to ensure you are doing the correct things at the correct time is paramount. Is it easy? Not always, but it sure beats years of discomfort and declining activity. I've heard of people who have suffered with tennis elbow for as long as 20 years.

As you'll learn, most elbow pain is due to damage of the soft tissues, rather than the bones. All tissues have the ability to heal over time. However, it's important to be doing the right things at the right time, in order to heal well. Unfortunately, most people don't do the right things at the right time in order to achieve the optimal healing and so set themselves up for recurring symptoms.

As I said earlier, there is always something that can be done. There are small changes that can be made, but you have to be ready to make that change. I have made suggestions to people in the past and have been met with resistance because they didn't want to make changes, or, better said, they didn't believe that small changes would make any difference, so they weren't willing to try. Doing nothing will never result in elbow pain completely resolving, it'll always come back, most likely a little bit worse and for a little bit longer each time.

"I'll have to take pain pills for the rest of my life." This action leads to wasted time, money and energy, not to mention the negative effects this can have on your body such as nausea, weakness and a weakened immune system [8.] Many people are thrilled to find that this statement is just not true. Pain pills are not great for your internal organs and being dependent on chemicals such as these is draining. There are many different options for pain relief and we will explore these later in the book.

6. You only get it in your dominant arm, but then it will spread to the other arm.

Most definitely not true. It all depends upon the overuse activity that caused the issue in the first place. Usually, people get Tennis Elbow in their dominant arm, due to repetitive motion and / or unaccustomed activities when they've been using their dominant arm more than usual or in a different way. I have seen many, many golfers who get tennis elbow, not golfer's elbow, but tennis elbow in their non-dominant arm. This is something to do with the biomechanics of the swing. Could it be due to the way they're gripping the club? Possibly. For example, I helped a lady who had developed tennis elbow in her non-dominant arm, by playing golf. You'll be happy to hear that she is back on the golf course and 100% pain free. More on her story later.

It could be that you are renovating your house and all of a sudden, you're spending hours and hours laying patio stones or with an electric drill in your hands. Maybe you are going to irritate that non-dominant side because it's not used to doing the things you are asking it to do. One client had been frantically cleaning her house before relatives came for the holidays and she was mopping all her floors and she got tennis elbow in her nondominant arm because it just wasn't used to doing so much activity all at once. So, you don't only get it in your dominant side.

No, it won't spread to the other arm. Do people get it on the other side, or even on both sides? Yes, they do. If someone delays getting the correct treatment, then unfortunately it is possible to develop similar symptoms in the other arm. The sooner you start doing the correct treatment, the sooner the symptoms settle down. The longer it's left, the more structures can be affected, and this is likely what leads to the other side developing issues.

What's going on there then if it does spread? A couple of different things. Let's investigate. Imagine you're right-handed and you're using your right hand all the time, for whatever repetitive motion it may be. Then you develop tennis elbow. Guess what, you're not going to use that arm. What are you going to do with the other side? You're going to do those repetitive motions with the other arm. Now, sometimes you can irritate the other side from that action. It can be a compensatory mechanism.

People who have suffered for a longer time, tend to have abnormalities in their shoulder and neck that can affect all the soft tissues of those areas too. It shouldn't be lost on you that there are some pretty major soft tissues coming out of the neck – the nerves. These can become affected in someone suffering with tennis elbow symptoms.

Imagine the nervous system as one continuous structure, from your brain, down your spinal cord with nerves exiting the spine at every single level. As one vertebra sits on top of another, there are small holes either side of the spine where the nerves come out and these nerves travel all the way down to the tips of your fingers or the tips of your toes. It seems logical to think that if one side of the nerve becomes irritated due to tennis elbow pathology, then it could affect the same nerve on the other side of the body. Hence symptoms can appear on the other side.

Let me put that another way. Tennis elbow is a tendon problem. Tendon problems are very closely related to nerve problems. The nerves come out of the neck and go down the arm and there are similar nerves that go down the other arm. If you irritate a tendon and a nerve on one side, it is likely that you will irritate a tendon somewhere else. Now it might not be a tennis elbow. It might be a golfer's elbow, a problem with the inside of the elbow. It might be a shoulder tendon. It might be a foot tendon or a knee tendon, but we know that if you have a tendon issue, many, many times the nerve is involved in some way. The nervous system becomes hyper-sensitized. This is the big picture that many healthcare professionals miss. Most of the time in people who are suffering with tennis elbow, a nerve will be irritated and if that nerve becomes hypersensitized other tendons can become affected too.

So, will it always spread to the other arm? No, but it can affect the other arm for some of the different reasons I mentioned above.

7. Anti-inflammatory medication will help as my elbow has been inflamed for months.

To investigate this myth, we must first understand how the healing process takes place. The healing process can be broken down into 3 distinct phases: the inflammation phase (the first

7 days after an injury), the repair phase (between 4 days and 2 months duration) and the remodeling phase (6 weeks to 12 months). [9, 10]

If the symptoms have been present for longer than a week, there are likely to be few inflammatory cells in or around the tendon. The way anti-inflammatory pills work is by reducing the inflammation, which in turn decreases symptoms. That is, you feel better. So, if there is not much inflammation at the tendon, there is not much for the anti-inflammatory pills to work their magic on and so symptoms remain unchanged.

It's important to say that now we understand the different phases of the healing process, it is possible to utilize anti-inflammatory medications in the event of an acute flare up. That would be, for example, if someone had been experiencing tennis elbow symptoms for 12 months, and we would recognize them to be in the remodeling phase of healing. However, if they were to undertake an out of the ordinary activity, such as moving to a new house; the heavy lifting, repeated motions, and consistent gripping of this activity may well irritate the tendon enough to cause an acute flare up of symptoms. Almost a new injury on top of an old one, if you like. This could be a potentially good opportunity for an anti-inflammatory medication to help reduce symptoms, as the acute phase of healing has been rekindled.

If you are in the very early stages of tennis elbow, meaning you've had symptoms for a few days, anti-inflammatories may help. If you've had this for three months, three years, or longer, anti-inflammatories are probably not going to make a whole lot of difference.

The reason for that is due to these stages of healing that we go through. When we have a soft tissue injury, the initial response is that the body sends inflammatory cells to the injured area to start the healing process. Now, if those inflammatory cells are there, anti-inflammatory medication can work on them and help to settle things down, but if you have had this for three months, three years, or longer, you are way past that initial phase of the healing process and so there are probably very few inflammatory cells there for your anti-inflammatory medication to work on. This is why anti-inflammatory medication is not going to work if you've had it for a long time. However, it can work in the early phases and it can also work if you flare up by doing something out of the ordinary.

Inflammation is the body's natural response to injury, and it has a set time frame. After 12 weeks, the inflammatory phase is absolutely over. So, why do some people still experience symptoms after 3 months?

The concept of chronic pain [11] has been around for many years now, but we still have much to learn. What we do know, is that when someone is still experiencing pain 3 months after an injury, or has symptoms that last longer than 12 weeks, the nervous system has become hypersensitized. This phenomenon can be resolved with targeted treatment. A skilled therapist can identify the causes of the symptoms that are still being felt. Often, this key part is missing from rehab and so people don't get better. I'll explain this concept in greater detail later in the book.

8. It's my age and my parents had it, so I guess it's going to be the same for me.

Tennis elbow is not a condition due to age. Granted, we absolutely do heal faster the younger we are, but tennis elbow isn't an age-related problem.

It is, however, a degeneration of the tendon, but not an aged-related degeneration like osteo-arthritis which is the wear and tear of the joints that everyone tends to get to a degree as we get older. To explain this, we need to back up a bit and learn a little bit about the anatomy of the area. A tendon is a connective tissue which attaches a muscle to the bone. That's all a tendon is, but, if a tendon becomes overworked, it will start to break down, that is, degenerate. This, degeneration of the tendon, is nothing to do with age though. Athletes and kids can get tennis elbow, just like anyone, if they overuse the tendon enough.

To give you a visualization of what happens during the degeneration of the tendon, imagine a tightly wound rope. This is what a normal tendon would look like if we did an ultrasound scan of it. Now, an ultrasound scan is different to ultrasound treatment that you may have heard about or even experienced. An ultrasound scan is the imaging they do for pregnant ladies when they get to see the baby. An ultrasound scan can be performed on soft tissues, such as on an elbow, so that the tissues inside can be seen.

If you did an ultrasound scan of a normal tendon, that tendon should look like a rope. All the fibers are very uniform, packed tightly together, and they are all in the same direction. That's what a normal tendon should look like on an ultrasound scan. If we do an ultrasound scan of an elbow that has tennis elbow, imagine that rope-like tendon unraveling. The fibers are no longer uniform or packed tightly together, but they are separated and haphazard. Cells can get in between the fibers, where they are not supposed to be and therefore cause irritation, weakness and other symptoms. That's what a degenerated tendon, or a tennis elbow tendon looks like on an ultrasound scan.

Despite this sounding maybe a little dramatic, there is good news. Recent developments in treatment techniques have resulted in much higher percentages of symptoms completely resolving. The ultrasound scans of these patients also show a reversal of the degeneration process [12.] It is not often that we can say that an issue can be reversed and completely resolved, but this is one of those times.

Here's a question I get asked really often: "I'm really frustrated that my elbow hasn't settled down this time as quickly as I thought it was going to, or as quickly as it has in the past. Is that because I'm getting older?"

There are a couple of different answers to this question. Is it that you're getting older? Well, we do heal more slowly as we get older, that is the case for sure. However, what tends to happen with episodic elbow pain is you experience a flare up of pain and it settles down. The next time it comes back, it's a little bit worse, but it'll settle down. The next time it comes back, it's a little bit worse again, it takes a little bit longer to settle down and then it'll settle down. The next time it comes back... This is what tends to happen, people get into this cycle.

So, yes, it will settle down, but if you don't do the correct things at the correct time, it will absolutely keep coming back. That's why I always stress to people that once we've got rid of the pain, if we don't do the other things that we need to do, like correct the movement patterns, get muscles stronger than they are right now, and stretch things out that are tight, it will absolutely keep coming back. It's very much an individual choice. To have elbow pain is not just part of aging. It's not something that everybody should have to put up with or experience.

Genetics can play a part in elbow pain, but there are many things that can be helpful. For example, my Grandad had a total knee replacement, and my Dad has also had a total knee replacement. Now that I know I have a genetic predisposition to osteoarthritis of the knees; I can take care of my knees. I just completed my second half marathon. Notice I said 'completed'. I didn't say I 'ran' my second half marathon. I know I can complete 13.1 miles comfortably if I use a combination of running and walking. If I try to run the whole way, I can only get to 10K (6 miles) before my knees start to tell me I'm going too far. Using that knowledge, I can modify my activity to preserve my knees but still participate in activities I love to do.

9. I need an x-ray or an MRI scan to see what's wrong.

Imaging for the elbow generally involves x-rays, MRI scans and maybe ultrasound scans. Are these procedures necessary for most people with elbow pain? No. So, why do so many people get irradiated, if it's not necessary? Surely, the doctor needs to see what's wrong with my elbow?

If you've had an x-ray, what did it show? Degeneration, bone spurs, joint disease, which are some scary words right there. But what do they mean? And is that what is causing your pain?

X-rays only show the bones. Therefore, unless you have a fracture in a bone, all the soft tissues; muscles, tendons, ligaments, nerves, don't show up on x-rays. Most people have no identifiable cause for their pain on x-ray [13.] Let's avoid unnecessary cost and radiation.

I'm currently in my 40s and I don't have elbow pain. Have I had it in the past? Yes, I have. I remember experiencing elbow pain when I was in my early 20s. This was when I was a newly qualified Physical Therapist, and I was working in a hospital with heavy patients. Have I suffered with episodic elbow pain since? No. I was lucky enough to be taught, by a great mentor of mine, how to do the right things at the right time and was able to heal my elbow effectively. Would you see a pristine elbow of a teenager if you took an x-ray of my arm? Heck, no. I'm in my 40s. You'd see the elbow of someone in their 40s, who also used to be a gymnast and dancer. My point is that everyone over the age of 30, is going to exhibit some aging of their joints on x-ray. That's normal. We all get it. Do those changes automatically lead to symptoms? No. Not if you take care of your body.

If you've had an MRI, what did it show? Degeneration, tendonitis, joint disease, but is that what is causing your elbow pain? MRIs are great because they show everything. MRIs are also not great because they show everything. MRI scans do show the soft tissues, but in most cases, the result of the MRI scan isn't going to change the treatment needed to resolve the cause of the problem. MRIs are costly and some people struggle with claustrophobia or panic attacks due to the confined nature of the procedure itself. Not a great situation.

If we do all the right things and we keep ourselves stretching and strengthening through the elbow, you can absolutely be completely pain-free, despite what your MRI may show or what your x-ray may show. I have thousands of clients that I've taken through this program and I know that I can get you to that point too.

10. Exercise will make it worse and I'm in too much pain to come to therapy.

The right exercise at the right time won't make it worse and will make it better. But do the wrong exercise and you may well increase your symptoms. Equally, doing the right exercise but at the wrong time can also make things worse. This is something I hear so often when people search YouTube for exercises to treat Tennis Elbow.

"I'm in too much pain to come to therapy," has to be my all-time favorite line. Please attend your therapy sessions especially if you are struggling. Therapy should not hurt you, and if it does, something is not right. There are many different strategies for pain relief. It can even be super helpful to attend therapy when you are really struggling, so that the therapist can identify exactly what is causing the problem and then administer treatment techniques for immediate relief and advise you on what to do, and not do, at home as well.

11. "I had physical therapy, and it didn't work."

This is my absolute, I was going to say favorite line, but it's not. When I hear people say they have tennis elbow and have tried physical therapy and it didn't work, it makes me really sad. Physical therapy absolutely does work, but only if you are doing the right things at the right time. That's the hardest part, and I get so frustrated. Physical therapy does work. My thousands of clients are testament to that. Physical therapy does work when it's done in the way it needs to be done. However, there is the issue that not all physical therapy is the same. Let me explain.

20 years ago, tennis elbow was treated as a standard soft tissue injury. Therapy would focus only on the involved elbow and about 50% of patients would recover from that episode. The 50% that didn't get better, would go on to have surgery and then 50% of them would improve. 50% would not. There were many "returners" to therapy, as the elbow would periodically flare up. Thankfully, now, with medical and scientific advances and research, those numbers can look very different. Every single person can make a complete and full recovery and return to everything they want to be doing, with no restrictions, but only if they do exactly what they need to do at the correct time. Individual guidance is essential.

Not all therapy clinics are created equally. Many patients

tell me how they have experienced other clinics, prior to finding me, where they were one of many people in a big room, where the therapist would spend a few minutes with them, before they were passed onto an unlicensed aide. Or were literally on a treatment conveyor belt, moving from one spot for heat, to another spot for stretching, then electrical stimulation or ultrasound and then ice. They would get the same treatment every time and the same treatment as everyone else. There was no individualization, no change in treatment plan depending on the patient's symptoms and no progression to ensure the problem didn't return.

I apologize to these patients, and I apologize to you if you have experienced this subpar version of therapy. How many people have experienced this and thought to themselves that physical therapy didn't work, so I must need surgery? It's my mission to save people from this fate. I'll now get down from my soapbox!

Would you go and see your primary care physician for an operation to repair a hole in your heart? No? Me neither. I'd want to go and see the cardiac specialist surgeon, preferably one who only does the procedure I needed. The point I'm trying to get across here, is that there is a massive difference between generalists and specialists. Most people know that MDs have different specializations, but did you know that that is also the case among many healthcare professions?

You may have been sent to the local general physical therapy clinic by your insurance or your family doctor when you needed some therapy. All PT is the same, right? Wrong. Just like specialist surgeons who have trained for years and then honed their skills during residencies and fellowships, on continuing education courses and under the guidance of mentors, physical therapists have too.

Physical therapists are the same in that, they're not all the same. I have coworkers and colleagues who are specialist physical therapists in the treatment of lymphedema. They work with cancer patients. I don't do that. That's not my specialty. I have physical therapy colleagues who work with pediatrics. They work with kids. That's not my specialty. I have physical therapy colleagues and coworkers that work with women's health, such as pelvic floor issues.

Whenever you have any kind of issue, you want to find a specialist for that issue. That is a reason general physical therapy doesn't work. They're the therapists who see two tennis elbows a year. They haven't got enough experience in healing tennis elbow. It's not their fault. They're too busy, treating all the backs and necks and knees and shoulders and everything else that comes through the door. But if you really want to get down to the core of the problem that you have and heal it properly, you need to work with the specialist. Physical therapy does work hands down. You've just got to find the right therapist.

That's why I recommend seeking out an experienced physical therapist who is specialized in treating tennis elbow. It does everyone a disservice if the therapist doesn't fully understand the complexity of the issue and how many different structures are potentially contributing to the symptoms. We can't just focus treatment on the elbow alone as that strategy rarely works. Unless all of the contributing structures are addressed the issue will definitely return or the poor patient will never feel relief in the first place, neither of which is an acceptable outcome. Just like you wouldn't see your general doctor to perform heart surgery on you, you would want to see the most specialized doctor focused on treating your specific issue. Specialists are naturally more skilled in their particular field, than their generalist peers. If you have Tennis Elbow, wouldn't you want to see the top specialist in that field? Someone who only helps people who have the same problem as you. A specialist will likely spend all of their time working with clients like you. A generalist may see someone with a problem like yours, but then they see someone with a neck issue, the next patient has a knee injury, then a sprained ankle comes hobbling in. Jack of all trades… I'll let you fill in the rest.

So, if you're looking for somebody that can help you on that journey and get you to the end destination of actually healing, not just get you pain-free, you've found the answer. If not, you know what? I'll see you in six months when your episode of pain comes back again.

Let's heal this elbow.

COVID-19 Update

Physical therapy is still a possibility due to technology and virtual visits. "How can you do physical therapy virtually? Don't you need to touch me?" This is a common misconception, and not just amongst clients, but within the physical therapist community too. When COVID-19 caused lockdowns around the world many physical therapy clinics closed their doors and haven't opened back up. When COVID-19 closed down my physical clinic location I immediately transitioned everyone to virtual visits. No-one went without treatment. I actually added services to keep our community healthy, boost immunity and prevent morbidity.

I have successfully rehabbed post-surgical clients, helped clients regain their mobility and independence, resolved ergonomic issues related to working from home, continued classes and added courses, all in the digital environment. I have helped more people, in more countries than ever before and my results are equivalent to my in-clinic results.

Most people can find relief after just one session, so, why then do people not do that? They are skeptical, I get it. When you've been let down by so many things you've tried before, you get to the point where you think nothing will work for you. You don't want to waste any more time and money on something else that will let you down. It's completely understandable. That's why a great strategy can be to search for success stories from people just like you. You can find many of my clients' success stories later in this book with snippets sprinkled throughout.

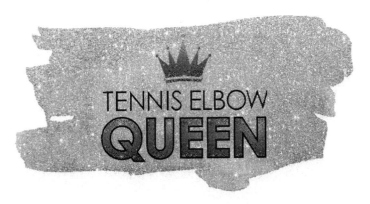

Success Story Snippet

66 Ultimately, Emma basically got me to understand how the body worked together. During the course of our time together I went from being unable to pick up that bottle of water I mentioned, to what I consider completely healed. My elbow gives me zero trouble anymore. It's now been eleven years since I saw her professionally, and she is still someone that I consider a very dear friend. If you are looking for someone that will take a real interest in your case, whatever your case may be, Emma is the only one that I would ever refer you to. Ever. She is phenomenal. Thanks, Emma. 99

– BG, male drummer, 30s, USA

CHAPTER 2

The Most Common Mistakes You Can Make If You Have Tennis Elbow

Doing Nothing

The biggest mistake has to be, doing nothing. Why suffer when you don't have to? This is a question I think about a lot. So many people have issues that could be helped really simply and even completely resolved with the right treatment. So, why don't they do it?

You might get to the point where you are so fed up with it hurting that you don't do anything. You don't play tennis. You don't play the musical instrument. You don't play with your kids. You don't lift your bag up when you go on the plane. You don't do all of these things because you know it's going to hurt. That's not living. That is not how it should be.

Maybe someone didn't know what to do, so they did nothing. Simply said, the person suffering didn't know there was a way to solve their problem. Maybe their doctor had told them that it was "Just their age" and "They had to live with it" or "Just take these pills". Maybe the surgeon had told them that surgery was the only option, but they didn't want to undergo such a drastic procedure, so accepted the fact that nothing could be done.

Please remember that there is always something that can be done. There actually may be several little things that can be done, which when added together can build to big changes over time. I guarantee there will be things I advise in my program that you won't have tried before. Have faith and trust the process. This has worked for thousands of people and can work for you, but only if you do it.

Pain Pills

Doctors and surgeons, by their very nature, are helpers. Everyone in the healthcare professions are helpers. If we weren't, we wouldn't last very long in the jobs that we do. Go and see a doctor with a problem and they want to help. They look in their "toolbox" and match something that can help you with your symptoms. For example, if you have pain, they may offer you a painkiller. If you have muscle spasm, they may offer you a muscle relaxer medication. If you have inflammation, they may offer you an anti-inflammatory pill. These tools can help, of course they can. Painkillers block the pain messages from getting through to your brain, where you would perceive it. But they don't heal the cause of the pain. Muscle relaxers can relax muscle spasm to allow you to feel much looser, until the medication wears off, and without healing the cause of the muscle spasm. Anti-inflammatory pills reduce inflammation because that's how they work to allow you to feel better. But they don't heal the cause of the inflammation.

These tools can be helpful during the healing process. For

instance, if you are unable to sleep due to pain, a medication can be helpful to allow you to get a good night's sleep. Sleep deprivation can be a form of torture, as any new parent would agree. We also heal when we sleep. So, if you can't sleep, guess what? No healing and big problem.

However, have you seen the side-effects? You look at the side of any bottle of medication and you can read about the side effects. What are you potentially doing to your liver, to your stomach, to your body? Thankfully, there are other ways to achieve a similar effect. We'll go through some examples later in the book.

Injections

Cortisone steroid injections used to be the go-to treatment for tennis elbow. You remember, I shared that my Mum had had 2. Thankfully, we now know that cortisone steroids can actually do more harm than good in soft tissue problems like tennis elbow. Cortisone can actually cause soft tissues to degenerate, as we learned in chapter 1. This is not a good situation. Thankfully, there are other options.

Platelet-rich plasma or PRP, is another type of injection that is popular among tennis elbow sufferers looking for relief. The research is not conclusive with regard to whether PRP can help tennis elbow heal or not. However, what I can tell you is that not all PRP is created equally. Many doctors offer PRP and the strength and type of PRP depends on the kit they have. How do you know which is the best for your particular problem? The answer is, you don't. It can be a shot in the dark, so to speak (excuse the pun). It may be prudent to avoid trying invasive procedures that are still being evaluated in the research.

Stem cell injections are another avenue being explored for

healing tennis elbow. This too is in the early stages of research. Therefore, the answer is we don't really know if it works. The same can be said for enzyme injections, vitamin injections, indeed, any kind of injections. Have you ever wondered why insurance companies don't cover these newer treatment techniques? It's because their effectiveness hasn't been completely demonstrated. As I mentioned above, thankfully injections are unnecessary in the treatment of healing tennis elbow.

Interestingly, I spoke with a client who had been in agony since a PRP injection 3 weeks prior. On chatting to him and trying to figure out exactly what was going on with him, it became apparent that the actual physical mechanism of the injection seemed to be the causative factor in his flare up. It was irrelevant to the substance that had been injected.

This anecdotal finding sits in line with research showing that patients who were suffering with tendon issues, who had multiple injections into the tendon, suffered for longer than those patients who didn't have injections, and had a worse outcome [6.] Thankfully, tennis elbow can be completely healed without injections of any kind.

Surgery

Go and see a surgeon with a problem and guess what they are going to do? They are going to look in their toolbox and see if they can offer you a solution to your problem. The best surgeons I work with, are the ones who turn patients away. Let that sink in for a moment.

These are the surgeons that will say "Surgery is not the right option for you. There are better options for your solution, but I don't have them." These surgeons refer patients to other healthcare providers for more conservative treatment. They may also only spend a really short amount of time with you, they are not being rude, they just know that they don't have the solution your problem needs. In other words, you're not their patient because you don't need surgery.

Go and see enough different surgeons, however, and you will find someone who will perform surgery on you. They may suggest a "Try it and see" surgery. I advocate a "Try everything else first and even then, get a second opinion if you need to" approach. Your body will thank you for it, like my husband thanked me.

In 2013, my husband thought he had stomach flu, but it gradually got worse until he ended up in Urgent Care. It was six days before Christmas and my son's kindergarten class was performing their Holiday Show, when I got a text from him, telling me that Urgent Care were referring him to the Emergency Room. I arranged for a friend to watch the kids and met him at the Emergency Room. The staff in the ER didn't know what was going on with my husband, so he was to be admitted for further investigations.

The following day my husband underwent a CT scan that came back inconclusive. He was steadily getting worse. They tried introducing a Nasogastric tube, which is a tube that goes up your nose and down your esophagus into the stomach, to see if they could release the pressure building in his abdomen. It didn't work. He continued to decline.

Three days before Christmas he called me early in the morning to say he was going into surgery. I called the hospital to speak with the surgeon as I was driving to drop the kids off with my friend. The surgeon I spoke with told me they still couldn't figure out what was wrong with my husband, so they were taking him to surgery, to open him up from his breastbone to his pubic bone, to see what was going on in there. He would then be transferred to Intensive Care, after such a major surgery. I asked the surgeon to wait until I got to the hospital, and he told me that we would not be able to delay the surgery for long.

When I arrived at the hospital, I was greeted at the door by a nurse who had been a previous patient of mine, "What are you doing here?" she cried. I was so relieved to see a familiar face and I relayed the situation to her and told her that we needed a second opinion. She anxiously looked at me as she said "But they're all away skiing." Don't ever get sick around the holidays. But she told me she would search and find me someone. I couldn't thank her enough.

She called my husband's internal medicine physician to come and speak with me and this was pivotal. He came in to see us and I asked him "If this was your son, what would you do?" This question allows the doctor to see your situation in a different light. You can see the change in their eyes. The internist looked at me intently and he said "I would wait until tomorrow. You have 24 hours." I sighed a huge sigh of relief that we had some time. The surgeon that the nurse had found for our second opinion came in and agreed that surgery was necessary, but that my husband should wait until the following day.

The next day my husband had his surgery laparoscopically (keyhole). He didn't need to spend any time in Intensive Care and was able to come home by the New Year. What a difference a day makes. My point is that, had I agreed to the solution the first surgeon had suggested, my husband would have had a vastly different experience. He would have been left with a 10-inch scar and been severely disabled for a period of time with a very lengthy recovery.

Now, I know that my husband's situation was an acute medical condition, which is quite different to a long-term chronic problem like tennis elbow, but the principle is the same, second opinions can be invaluable. Surgeons, doctors and other healthcare professionals offer different options for the same problem. The challenge the patient has is knowing which option to choose. Getting more than one opinion can be a way to help. Also, trying all conservative options, before starting with invasive options, is generally the best way to proceed.

Brace / Strap / Clasp

There are so many different devices marketed to Tennis Elbow sufferers. New ones come out all the time. One client I know is still searching for the brace that's going to work for him and he's already got five in his closet. He has spent over $800 on just one. He's searching for the magic brace that's going to make his elbow better. But guess what? It is not there.

Braces or straps can take pressure off the tendon, but once you put something external on your arm, the muscles will switch off. This is a big issue for full healing. Let me explain. When your elbow started to hurt, you will have changed the way you do things to try to prevent the pain. By doing this, you will have stopped using your arm to a degree. Whenever we stop using a muscle, it starts to waste within hours.

One study found a decrease in protein synthesis after just 6 hours of immobilization [14]. Protein is the substance that muscles are made from and as we use our muscles, the protein is consistently replenished. If protein stops being made in the muscles, that's going to cause wasting pretty quickly. Another study showed that muscle fiber size had decreased by 17% in just 72 hours of immobilization [15]. That's the wasting we were talking about. Another study showed that immobilizing the forearm for just 9 days caused a 32.5% decrease in strength [16]. Imagine how much strength could be lost after 9 weeks, 9 months or 9 years. A similar study found that it took women longer to regain their strength, than their male counterparts [17.] These studies were done on healthy, uninjured individuals who had casts placed on their wrists.

So, we know that by using a brace or strap, the muscles will waste. Part of the problem of tennis elbow is that the muscles are weak. Phase 3 of my program is strengthening, which is essential as this is when we actually heal the tendon. But relying on a brace or strap will accentuate the weakness and therefore, prevent the healing from occurring, which is not a good outcome.

My advice is not to use a brace or a strap if you can help it. There may be times when you need one, such as moving to a new house, which I mentioned in the previous chapter as something that can lead to flare-ups in elbows, or you may be in a job where you have to use your arms and can't rest. I had a client who was a sushi chef and just couldn't change the way he worked and couldn't slow down either. A strap was invaluable to allow him to continue his work and be able to feed his kids. A recent study showed that sufferers who wore a wrist brace benefited from some pain relief [37.] Just don't become reliant on a strap or brace. Our ultimate goal is to wean you off and get you back to doing all the things you want to do with no restrictions.

Rest

If someone sees you struggling with something, what do they say? "Take it easy." If someone sees you in pain, what do they say? "Rest it." These are the right things to do, but only for the first 3 days after an injury. After that point, the tissues are starting to heal and need normal stresses and strains to go through them in order to heal in a strong and efficient way.

But how do you know that it's safe to move? A Licensed Physical Therapist is a movement and injury specialist who has the knowledge and expertise needed to guide you through the healing process. As we've just learned the longer you defer getting back to doing your normal activities, the more the muscles will weaken. The more the muscles weaken, the harder it is to get back to doing all the things you love.

There are so many options to try, but which are the right ones for you? That's the challenge right there. Some people need one particular thing and some need the exact opposite. How would you know which options are safe and effective for you to try? The good thing is, there are some helpful tips that you can start from today, that are safe for all. I'll walk you through these later in the book.

Exercises From YouTube

YouTube has a lot of answers, but you need to ensure that the answers you find are the answers to the questions you are asking. Better said, you need to know what you are searching for before plugging something like "Exercises for Tennis Elbow" into the search bar of YouTube. Wondering why? Go on. Try it. Right now. Let's see what comes up.

You back? Well... what did you find? A ton of exercises for tennis elbow, right? Yes, there's certainly a lot of advice out there. However, how do you know which are the right exercises to heal your elbow? You don't know. I can tell you that there is some great advice out there and there's also some that will absolutely make you worse. So, what should you do? If you're like most people, you probably get completely overwhelmed by the amount of differing advice and so do nothing. Understandably so. You don't want to try something that might make it worse, and so it feels safer to stick with the status quo.

What if you're one of the people that found one of the videos that had a lot of views and some good comments under it. Narrowing it down like that makes sense. So, you try what they suggest, and it makes it hurt like heck. What do you do now? Is it supposed to feel like that? Who can you ask? Silence. So, you stop doing the new exercise and stick with what you know, which is sensible.

You can find videos that say "This is the best exercise for tennis elbow. Here's what you've got to do and that's going to cure you". Unfortunately, that's highly unlikely. Which phase of healing are you in? What other symptoms have you got? What other structures are involved? Are they going to get you better? No, they're probably not because they're probably not the right exercises or you might not even be doing them correctly.

Can you get the exercises you need from YouTube? No. This assumes that tennis elbow is a simple condition that needs a simple solution to resolve it. This is absolutely not the case. Tennis elbow is a multi-faceted condition that can affect many different structures, which I'll explain in more detail later in the book. But the multi-faceted nature of this condition requires a much higher level of understanding to fully heal it so that it never comes back. If you don't address every aspect of your tennis elbow, you will not resolve it completely and it will return.

Massage

Is massage going to help? Yes, generally it is. Is massage going to cure tennis elbow? No, it isn't. Not by itself. Do you need to go and see a massage therapist? Only if you want to, but you don't have to as you can do the soft tissue treatment techniques that you need at home. You don't need somebody else to do that for you. Your elbow is a very accessible part of your body. You can get to it yourself. I'll teach you what you need to do later in the book.

Ultrasound And Other Electrotherapy

I can't remember the last time I used ultrasound. Ultrasound was something that I learned to do a long time ago when I was in physio school. It does have a place with certain conditions and at certain times within those conditions. But is ultrasound going to help tennis elbow? No, it's not. So, you don't need to search out somewhere to have ultrasound treatment.

Oh, and by the way; you can take "ultrasound" out and you can put "laser" in there. You can take "laser" out and you can put "interferential" in there. You can take "interferential" out and you can put "EStim" in there. None of these electrical modalities heal tennis elbow [18.]

A relatively new modality is extracorporeal shock wave therapy. I have never actually experienced this but have heard from people who have tried it that it's pretty painful. There was lots of buzz about it healing tennis elbow – you may even have heard this yourself. Unfortunately, the research shows that it is not beneficial in the treatment of tennis elbow [19.]

I learned how to do infrared in physio school and I never used it on a patient. Infrared is essentially just heat. I'm hearing about infrared saunas and all the benefits that they have right now and infrared lamps. Do you need to run out and buy one? No, you don't. It's not going to give you any more benefit than a hot water bottle or a heating pad or a hot towel or a hot shower. Please do not feel you have to do and spend money on these things because you think that's the thing that's going to make you better. It's not. You can get some great relief from things you already have around the house.

Keep reading to learn which strategies to start with and how to apply them.

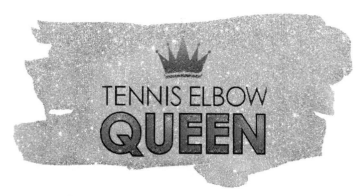

Success Story Snippet

❝I wish somebody had told me back when I first got injured, that you need to be looking for somebody who will both prioritize your recovery, as well as your success thereafter. That it's not just let's get you fixed, let's put a band aid on it and make it so that you can just function, but someone who will make sure that I can function, but then also thrive afterwards. That I can chase my goals, that I can be as athletic and as ambitious as I want to be. And that it's not just okay, now you can carry things. It's okay you can carry things, you can do pull-ups, you can do a stunt show, you can keep training, you can go back to kickboxing, like it doesn't matter.**❞**

– SB, active female, 20s, USA

CHAPTER 3

Why Did You Get Tennis Elbow?

Why did you get tennis elbow? Why do people get tennis elbow? There are a few different reasons, let's explore each one in turn.

Overuse

The most common and the number one cause of tennis elbow is overuse [20.] Whenever I start working with a new client, one of the first questions I ask them is, "How long have you been suffering?" Now regardless of how long they've actually had it (I do need to know this to effectively plan their treatment program) I want to know what changed three to six months before they started feeling their symptoms. Something changed.

Did you start a new workout regime? Did you start doing new exercises? Did you increase the weight on certain exercises? Sometimes it can be that. Did you start a new activity? Did you take up tennis? Did you renovate your house? Did you go traveling? Has your work set-up, your workstation changed? Many people right now are working from home and that's a huge change. Instead of their wonderful standing desk and ergonomic chair at work, they are now sitting on a kitchen or a dining room chair at the table. This can cause a change in stresses and strains around the elbows and can irritate tendons and other soft tissues.

Have you spent time painting your garden fence? What have you been doing that flared this up? There's likely some kind of overuse problem in your history. Now, the reason that we want to try and find out what it was, is so that we can stop doing it or change it or make it into a much kinder activity for the elbow. There are ways to change activities. It's not always about completely stopping something. It can be a change and that's why we want to figure out what's caused it.

- **Stop and have a think right now:**

When did my elbow pain start?

_____

_____

_____

What was the date 3 months before this?

_____

_____

_____

What was the date 6 months before this?

_____

_____

_____

What was I doing around those times?

_____

_____

_____

Hopefully, you may have uncovered what caused your elbow pain. If not, let's read on.

Altered Biomechanics

The second cause can be altered or abnormal biomechanics. Many times, when we think about biomechanics, sports jump immediately to mind. We may think about tennis. We may think about golf. We think about these different sports that people enjoy, and we look at how people move as they're doing these different activities.

But biomechanics is not always a sport related thing. It could be the way you're painting your garden fence. You could be using an abnormal biomechanical movement to do that, abnormal for you that is. Maybe you're holding the brush in an awkward way. Maybe there's a problem with your shoulder that's having a knock-on effect in your elbow and we delve into the causes of this issue below. Or maybe it could be overuse because you've been doing it for hours and hours and hours on end.

Maybe it was just the technique or the way you were doing it. Maybe you had an injury to your shoulder, so you've changed the way you move and do things. It can be something as simple as that. We want to try and pull out what was the cause and the reason behind it.

Direct Trauma

The third cause can be a direct injury. Tennis Elbow tends to be an overuse issue, but not always. I have seen clients who have slipped, tripped, or bumped their elbow right on the tendon and created an inflammatory reaction that then led to tennis elbow. That's how a direct injury can cause tennis elbow. It is much less common, but it does happen. Thankfully, the same strategies work to settle it down, regardless of the cause.

Compensation Mechanism

The fourth cause can be as a compensation mechanism for another injury. As I alluded to with the biomechanics, if you've hurt your shoulder, you're using your arm in a different way and you irritate the elbow. Maybe you have broken your wrist and you can't use that arm. All of a sudden, the other arm's doing all the work and so you irritate the tendon. It can be as a consequence of another injury. Indeed, a study done in the UK found a high correlation of tennis elbow in people who had a history of rotator cuff issues in their shoulder, carpal tunnel syndrome or a De Quervains problem in the thumb [21.]

Antibiotics

One cause of tendon problems that a lot of people don't know about is this one, which is taking certain antibiotics [22.] It is a rare cause of tennis elbow, but it can happen. If people do suffer with tendon issues caused by taking antibiotics, it tends to lead to Achilles tendon problems, but other tendons can also be affected. I know a handful of clients who developed tennis elbow in this way. So, sometimes it can be that when we're looking for a cause. If I ask, "What happened?" and they respond with "I can't think of anything. Oh, wait, I had a chest infection and I had to take antibiotics for it." Maybe that's it. It can be.

Ergonomics

Poor ergonomics is another contributing factor that we look for. I alluded to this a little earlier on when I mentioned workstation setup. Our bodies are designed to be in a nice upright, straight position. Think about your ear lobe, shoulder and hips all being nicely aligned when we're standing or sitting. That's where our spine and bodies like to be.

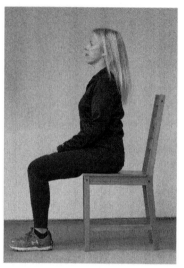 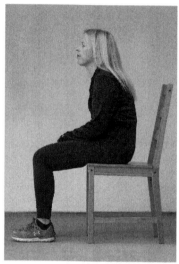

However, most people adopt a "C" shaped curve in their spine when they're working on their computer, especially if they're working on a laptop.

That "C" shaped curve puts a lot of pressure on your spine, especially your neck. It can put a lot of pressure on the nerves that come out of the neck and go all the way down to the tips of your fingers. There is a big correlation between tendons and nerves. If you irritate a nerve or pinch a nerve, that can cause a tendon to become inflamed. We'll delve deeper into the causes and the importance of this in the next chapter.

Therefore, there are several reasons that people get tennis elbow, but thankfully, the strategies to heal it are all similar. But what exactly IS tennis elbow? Read on my friend, read on.

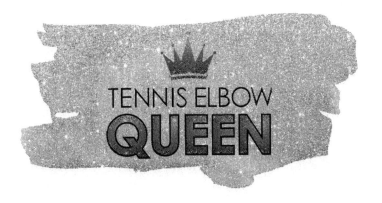

Success Story Snippet

❝I'm so grateful for having found Emma when I did, and enrolling on to her elbow programme; it quickly put my mind in a more positive space with the light at the end of the tunnel that I needed to focus on. After just a month on the course, I was mostly pain free day to day, and after 3 months I gradually started getting back to the things I love doing.**❞**

– WH, active male, 20s, UK

CHAPTER 4

What's Tennis Elbow?

've spent all this time talking to you about tennis elbow, well what is it? The little sub-heading I like to put under here is "When an **'itis'** isn't inflammation". Now, obviously the term Tennis Elbow doesn't have that "itis" in it, but lateral epicondylitis is the medical terminology for tennis elbow. Lateral, meaning on the outside. So, the outside of the elbow is where we get tennis elbow, the inside is where people get golfer's elbow.

The lateral epicondyle is the bony point on the outside of the elbow, probably where it's a little tender, that's your lateral (outside) epicondyle of the elbow. This is where the tendon that is affected by tennis elbow attaches. This is the common extensor tendon. Basically, the common extensor tendon becomes unhappy.

Let's go into a little bit of anatomy. Firstly, let's consider the bones. There's the long bone that comes down from the shoulder to the elbow. That's called the humerus. Then there are two bones that create your forearm, the radius and the ulna. On the outside of the elbow, the bony point is called the lateral epicondyle. This is where the common extensor tendon attaches.

Tendons basically attach muscles onto bones. The muscles of your forearm, which make your hand go up from the wrist, are attached onto that bony part, the lateral epicondyle, which is that bone on the outside of the elbow, by the common extensor tendon.

Muscle is a very stretchy tissue. It's designed to contract and relax to move. But the muscle is attached onto the bone by a tendon. A tendon is essentially a connective tissue. It connects the muscle to the bone. It is not as stretchy as muscle, just a little bit stretchy.

Epicondylitis is a medical term, where "-itis" means inflammation in Latin. Hence epicondyl- refers to the epicondyle and it is, meaning inflammation, or inflammation of the epicondyle. Earlier, we learned that anti-inflammatories don't often work on tennis elbow, or lateral epicondylitis, and the reason for that is because the inflammatory response, the inflammation, the "itis", only occurs in the very early phase of tennis elbow. Once you get past the first three weeks, there really is not much inflammation there [9, 10] unless you've irritated it. So, lateral epicondylitis is not really a good descriptive name for this problem, unless you've had it for a very short amount of time, or have recently irritated it, in which case it would absolutely apply.

You may hear the term lateral epicondylopathy; meaning lateral (on the outside), epicondyl- (the bony bit of the elbow), opathy, means pathology. Essentially, there's something going on with the outside of your elbow, is what that means. It's very much an umbrella term that we use because we don't know if it's an "itis". Sometimes you might hear "tendinosis". "Itis" means acute inflammation or a problem that you've not had for very long. "Osis" means chronic or a problem that's been hanging around for a while. So, "tendinopathy" covers everything. But with good old tennis elbow, you know what you're talking about. It's all the same thing.

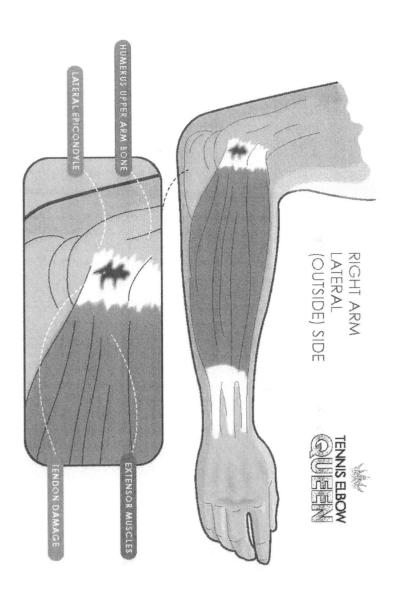

In tennis elbow it is that tendon that becomes unhappy, so it's not a muscle tear. It's not a muscle problem per se. The tendon that attaches the muscle onto the bone is the tissue that is affected. In the very early stages of this problem, that is, in the first few days, you might have some inflammation going on. After that, you likely don't have much, unless you irritate it specifically.

Why then, do I still feel pain? Great question. The answer is because the tendon is degenerating. This is a degeneration that has nothing to do with age. When we hear the word "degeneration", we imagine we are falling apart. But this degeneration of the tendon has nothing to do with age. It's all to do with the pathology and that's what causes the irritation that the tendon is susceptible to.

The reason that tennis elbow can last so long is that tendons have an extremely poor blood supply. In the picture you can see the muscle is shaded in. Muscles have a great blood supply because they need lots of oxygen coming in to let them work and move. Tendons, as you can see in the picture, are shaded white because they don't have a very good blood supply. It's just essentially a connective tissue that attaches the muscle onto the bone. So, it doesn't need a lot of blood supply to do that job. However, it does need a good blood supply to heal itself and tendons don't have a good blood supply and that's the reason they take so long to heal.

Therefore, we want to try and increase the circulation to the area. The body is an amazing thing. The body recognizes that it needs to get more blood flow into the tendon to heal it. It recognizes that there's not enough blood flow going into the tendon. So, the body grows new blood vessels into the tendon to try and get more blood to it. The body is really trying to heal itself. It grows new vessels in there to get more blood to the area in order to heal it. This is not normal. The tendon shouldn't have these new blood vessels in it. The body is really trying to heal itself. I mentioned that ultrasound scans can be a great way to view the tendon. There's also a type of ultrasound scan that can view blood vessels. Therefore, if we see these additional blood vessels on an ultrasound scan as well, it's part of the pathology and is called neovascularization; "neo" meaning new and "vascularization" meaning blood vessels [23].

Years ago, basic therapies were used to treat tennis elbow and about half of patients would feel better afterwards. However, if you did an ultrasound scan of their elbow, the tendon would still look degenerated. The tendon did not change. Symptoms settled down, so the patient felt better, but it didn't truly heal and that's why it would come back because the tendon was still degenerated.

Thankfully, we've known about more effective types of treatment techniques for over 20 years. With these newer ways of healing tendons, essentially, we don't just settle the symptoms, we change the tendon. That's how we know the degeneration that occurs in tennis elbow is not due to aging. For example, you could take an x-ray of my spine and you would see wear and tear changes. In everybody over the age of 30, you will see wear and tear changes in the spine if you take an X-ray. It's essentially normal. We all get it. That's aging degeneration. That's not reversible at the moment. Who knows in the future? But right now, that is not reversible.

We do know that the degeneration of a tendon affected by tennis elbow can change. That's what the newer treatment techniques do. They change the degeneration so that if you did an ultrasound scan of that elbow once it is healed, imagine seeing that rope tightened back up again, like it should be. The thickened injured tendon returns to a more normal size [24]. It's truly amazing what the body can do. It can heal itself with the right environment, and by doing the right things at the right time. Essentially what I'm saying is tennis elbow can be completely, absolutely, 100% resolved.

Why It Can Last So Long

Why do some people suffer with this for such a long time if we know that tennis elbow can be completely resolved? If somebody's had tennis elbow for several years, not only is it affecting the tendon, it's affecting other structures too. It's like a ripple effect. If you drop a pebble into a pond, you get the ripples spreading out. If the elbow is where your problem started, the longer you have it, the larger the ripple effect is going to spread. It's going to affect the forearm muscle. It's going to affect the biceps muscle. It's going to affect the shoulder joint. It's going to affect your shoulder blade. It's going to affect your neck. It's going to affect your wrist and hand.

The longer you've had tennis elbow, the more tissues are going to be involved and they all need addressing because they will not be functioning correctly. They will not be receiving their normal neural input, which are basically messages from the nerves. They're not getting the correct messages from the nerves because of the pathology that has been going on for such a long time. This can all be resolved too, but it needs addressing in order to settle down. These are the other issues that many times are not addressed.

If you go to see somebody and say, "I have tennis elbow, I've had it for three years" and they say, "Let me look at your elbow". Okay, that's a great start and can confirm the diagnosis, but that's likely not the whole story. If you don't settle all those other structures down, your elbow pain will come back. If you just focus treatment on the elbow and you don't work on everything else that has been affected by that prolonged tennis elbow, the issue will come back every time. Unfortunately, that's why people say physical therapy doesn't work. "Oh, I tried. It didn't work for me." Well, that's probably why. Everything needs to be addressed and then this can be completely settled down once and for all so that it does not come back, and you are able to do everything you want to do with no restrictions whatsoever.

What Is Pain?

Pain is a sensation perceived in the brain. It can indicate tissue damage, for example picking up a hot pan, OW. Your brain perceives the intense heat through your tissues and sends a message down to your hand to "Let go." But does pain always mean tissue damage? No, not always. Try this out, right now; pull your little finger back as far as it can go. Now push it just a little further, OW. Your body is warning you to not push any further, or tissue damage will happen. This is a protective mechanism.

Then, if I'm feeling pain, I shouldn't push through, right? As in a few answers I give, it depends. If you've just injured yourself, as in it's really recent, within 3 days, then "No", you shouldn't push it. But if you were injured over 3 months ago, then you are safer to push. A Licensed Physical Therapist can guide you through this situation. Their knowledge of tissue healing at particular time frames will allow them to make the best selection of treatment options at each particular stage.

Chronic Pain

Chronic pain is a situation that can develop after someone has been feeling pain for over 3 months. Not everyone develops chronic pain, and we don't know why some people do and some people don't, but we are learning more about chronic pain all the time. Chronic pain is real. Not that long ago, people who suffered from chronic pain were told that it was all in their head.

Ironically, to a degree, we've discovered that that is true, as when chronic pain occurs, there are physiological and anatomical changes to the brain [25.] Chronic pain is a cycle that leads the nervous system to become hypersensitized [26.] This means that it doesn't take much to trigger a nerve. Let me explain that a little further.

All nerves are stimulated by certain sensations, for example, touch. When does a firm touch, such as a handshake, become painful like a pinch? Your nervous system delivers the information on how hard, or soft, the pressure is. Now imagine your nervous system is hypersensitized, and now that firm handshake feels like a pinch, OW. The nervous system is sending too many messages, too quickly, and the person feels way more than they should due to the level of pressure being applied.

Thankfully, there are treatment techniques that can normalize the nervous system. This is one of the most common missing links I see in the treatment of Tennis Elbow. 95% of the Tennis Elbow clients I see have some sort of nerve involvement in their problem. Be sure to ask your healthcare provider about how they will address the issue of the hypersensitized nervous system. In my experience, if the nervous system is not addressed correctly, the problem is not truly resolved and will return.

How do you know if you have nerve involvement? What do nerve symptoms feel like? Pain, electric shocks, tingling, pins and needles, numbness, ants crawling on the skin, water trickling; I've had clients use all these descriptions. I had a new client today describe "Knives" in her arm. Can you relate to some of these symptoms?

What causes it? There are a number of different problems that can cause nerve symptoms, so what works for one person, may not work for another if the cause of their symptoms is different. Makes sense, right? Nerve symptoms can be caused by pressure on the nerve from an internal structure such as a bulging or herniated disc in the spine, an inflamed or arthritic joint in the neck, a tight muscle in the shoulder or forearm, pressure on the nerve from an external source like a hard table or arm rest or shortening of the nerve due to a muscle imbalance or not using the arm normally. As you can see, there's a lot to investigate with nerve symptoms, which an experienced practitioner can test and talk you through.

The nerve itself can become irritated. A nerve is a soft tissue like a muscle or a ligament. Soft tissues can shorten and tighten. They adapt to the stresses and strains that we're putting through them. For example, if you've not stretched out your pecs for a long time and you do lots and lots of work on building up those muscles, but you don't stretch them out, they're going to get tight. Similarly, with a nerve, if you're not stretching a nerve out, and you're not mobilizing a nerve, it can become tight, and you can get a tension within the nerve itself that can then become irritated and uncomfortable.

Why Do Anything About A Bit Of A Niggle?

Why do people have this problem when they shouldn't? People put things off. We're all guilty of it. Guess how long it took me to write this book! Sometimes when we put things off, it can have a detrimental effect on us and our quality of life. If someone went to see a Licensed Physical Therapist, with a bit of a niggle in their elbow, it would be pretty straightforward to figure out what would be the best course of action for that person, get them doing the right things, prevent it from getting worse and alleviate it.

I will tell you, that rarely happens. Most people wait until they can't take it any longer or are unable to pick up the crying baby in the middle of the night, or until the rip-roaring pain has them sobbing to their spouse at 3 o'clock in the morning, or, when the nerve pressure becomes nerve damage, and they lose their strength. Guess how much longer these issues take to settle down? So much longer. However, that's human nature, where we put off things until we absolutely have to deal with them. If you have a bit of a niggle at the moment, do yourself a favor and get it looked at now. Imagine the heartache, pain, time, energy and money you'll be saving yourself and your family.

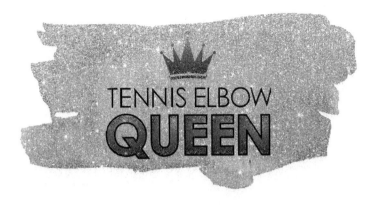

Success Story Snippet

❝I am back playing tennis, which for a while there I was wondering when and if that would ever happen. I was out for 11 months, and for six of those, I was with Emma and she got it done.❞

– PL, male tennis player, 50s, USA

CHAPTER 5

Why Do You Need A Guide?

Why do you need a guide? I guess that's the big question, isn't it? "Emma, can't I get all the information off the internet?" Well, yes and no. Most of the information that I gathered over the past 13 years, whilst I was working with my clients and collating it into the program that I now deliver, is all out there. It's not rocket science. The information is all out there, but you've got to know where to look and, more importantly, you've got to know how to apply it. You've got to know what's good information and what's not.

You've also got to know which phase of healing you are in right now. If you're reading this book, you're more than likely going to be in phase one, but what does that mean and why does it matter? Let me explain about the four phases to heal your elbow.

Phase 1

Phase one is when you are feeling the symptoms. It's uncomfortable, and you can't sleep at night. You can't do things. You can't pick up a cup of coffee or a bottle of water without feeling pain. Phase one treatment settles down the symptoms. It gets rid of the sharp discomfort. It begins to relax the muscle tension that you've got. It just starts everything feeling a bit more back to normal. Once you've got yourself into a routine with phase one, you can move into phase two.

Phase 2

Phase two is about normalizing the soft tissues and regaining range of motion if you've lost any. Now that is not necessarily range of motion in the elbow. It may be range of motion in the neck. It may be range of motion in the shoulder or the shoulder blade, depending on how things are moving. But phase two covers regaining range of motion and normalizing soft tissues. It's very much about addressing the tissue tightness, the forearm tightness, upper trapezius (shoulder stress muscles) tightness. Getting things moving normally helps to get things feeling much more normal. There's quite a bit of overlap from phase one to phase two and together, they can start helping fast.

Phase 3

Phase three is my favorite phase, it's all about strengthening. You will have weakened muscles if you have been suffering with tennis elbow. The reason for this is that it hurts, so you're not going to use your arm as much as you would normally do. As soon as we stop using something, it starts to weaken. We learned about that in chapter 2.

You will have muscle weakness as part of your tennis elbow, and it is something that needs to be addressed. We need to strengthen everything back up. There are different ways of strengthening. There is a way that will irritate you and there's a way that will heal you. The magic happens when you know which is which. It depends on your symptoms. It depends on your situation. It depends on the phase that you're in. I will guide you through this.

Phase 4

Phase Four is going to be your favorite as you'll get back to doing everything you want to do. It'll get you back to playing tennis, playing golf, running, biking, cycling, rowing, working out, playing the drums, playing the guitar, playing the violin and the viola, swimming, picking your kids up, picking up the groceries, renovating your house, using a screwdriver, all of those things that you can't do right now; even picking up that glass of water, or that cup of coffee. It gets you back to doing everything you want to do with no restrictions.

Which Phase Are You In?

Which of the 4 phases are you in; one, two, three, or four? (There's a quiz that can tell you from your symptoms. Access it in the book bonuses:

http://bit.ly/TE-bookbonuses

How do you know which phase you're in? Which exercises, which advice, what do you need to be doing for each of those phases? The information is all out there. Will you find it packaged neatly, so you can understand it? Probably not. If you've ever read a research article and particularly a medical research article, they're pretty dry (there are many listed at the end of this book). There are not many pictures and they're quite repetitive. The outcome of all of them is that more research is needed because it always is. We are always learning. That's why my program evolves over time. I change things as new research comes out.

I can guide you through this process. I've been helping clients for the past 13 years, and my program is successful. It's really successful. I love helping people. I love seeing the change on their faces as they start to feel better. So many people when they first start working with me, have a pained look on their faces, like they are right at the end of their tether. They've tried everything. The most memorable are the people who have tried everything before; they've got the brace, they've done ice, they've been to PT and they end up sitting in front of a surgeon and saying, "I want surgery".

This is exactly what had happened to my very first client. I'll tell you his story and you can hear him tell his story here:

http://bit.ly/TE-bookbonuses

because he tells it so much better than I do and he's more than happy for me to share his story, so I share this a lot.

The very first client that I healed actually came to me by default. Let's go back 13 years in time. 13 years ago, I was working at my local hospital as a physical therapist in outpatients, seeing everybody, backs, necks, shoulders, knees, a little bit of everything. By chance, I shared an office with an occupational therapist and another physical therapist. At the end of every day, we would write our notes up together, we got on really well, and it was a fun office.

One day the occupational therapist was writing her notes and she put her notes down, sat back in her chair, looked at me and said, "I've got this patient". You always know that you're going to get a story when somebody says that. So, I put my pen down and I sat back to listen. She told me about her client. He'd searched for help everywhere around California. He had seen everyone around Los Angeles. He was a professional drummer, and he couldn't drum because he had tennis elbow. So, he ended up sitting in front of the surgeon and he said to her, "I've been everywhere. I've tried everything. I'm a professional drummer and I can't drum. Give me surgery on this elbow so I can drum."

This is why I love the surgeon I work with. She said, "No, I don't know exactly what treatment you've tried up to now, so I want you to go and see my therapists at the hospital first." He was upset as he said, "I want surgery, I need this fixed now." She said, "I'm not going to do anything until you go see them. I don't know who you've seen and what they've done. You need to go and see my people first. Then, if you still have problems, come back to see me." He wasn't happy at having to wait longer, but he did set up the appointment with the occupational therapist, who the surgeon wanted him to see.

So, my friend, the occupational therapist, had treated him for a few sessions for his elbow. He was asking all kinds of different questions, he was saying to her, "Do you think my thoracic spine can have an effect on my elbow? I read somewhere that if you treat the thoracic spine, it can help tennis elbow." The thoracic spine is the mid back. My occupational therapist friend is a Certified Hand Therapist. She is one of the most knowledgeable, experienced, amazing therapists I've ever worked with. She deals with clients who have shoulder, elbow, wrist, and hand problems. She helps people from the shoulder down. She doesn't deal with the spine. So, this was her question to me. She said, "I have this patient who's tried all these things. He's asked me about treatment for his thoracic spine. What do you think?"

I knew that for sure, the cervical spine (the neck) can affect the elbow, but I wasn't sure about the thoracic spine. So, I said, "Put him on my list. Let me see him."

So, we met, and I think he probably rolled his eyes again; somebody else, yet another pair of eyes looking at him. I worked with him over a period of months and we peeled back the layers of what needed addressing. He was right. He did need work on his thoracic spine, as well as his neck, his shoulder blade, his shoulder, his upper trapezius muscle, and his elbow, wrist and hand, plus the nerves that go down his arm. He needed everything. So, we went through and addressed everything.

This included coming up with a new way of treating tennis elbow, to ensure that it fully healed once and for all. He would do the exercises himself at home and integrate the other strategies that I had added to address all the different elements of his issue. Within 6 months, he was able to get back to playing the drums. All these years later, he's still doing great. His tennis elbow completely resolved. He continues to play drums, he writes music, he is successful, and he is pain free. Did he need surgery? No. Did he need injections? No. So, I tell you this story to know that there is hope when you find the right person who has the solution to the problem that you have. You've found your guide. I can take you through this. So, let's begin our journey.

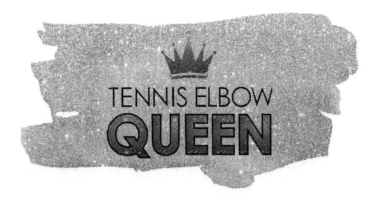

Success Story Snippet

Newly retired lady who loved playing golf developed tennis elbow in her non-dominant arm after increasing the number of days per week she was out on the golf course. After completing the Tennis Elbow Relief program, she was pain free and able to play golf as much as she wanted with no restrictions.

– JL, female golfer, 60s, USA

CHAPTER 6

Phase 1
Self-Help Strategies

The Power Of The Right Solution

What can you do to help? This section contains all the self-help strategies that I share in Phase 1 of my online Tennis Elbow Relief Program. Find out more about my comprehensive program here:

http://bit.ly/TE-bookbonuses

Every single strategy can be started today, right now at home with minimal equipment. There's a lot that you can do to help and we're going to go through each and every action item in detail.

Heat The Heck Out Of It

The first thing that I recommend to all my clients is heat. Heat is your friend. "But Emma, I thought I was supposed to put ice on my elbow." Or people say, "Well, how do I know whether to put ice or whether to put heat? Which should I do? Is it this one? Is it that one or not? I don't know." Great questions!

Generally, if it is very acute, maybe you have been pulling up weeds all day because it was a nice day outside and you've been out in the garden, pulling weeds and your elbow's really flared up, ice your elbow. If you have any acute injury, then you need three days of ice. But you can still heat your neck, heat your shoulder and your forearm. We want to get heat into these tissues to relax the muscles off.

You're going to need a heating pad, a hot towel or a hot water bottle. I know many of you will probably stand a little bit longer under a hot shower, just because it feels good. Heat of any source can work. I recommend heating pads just because they tend to be a little easier to use throughout the day. There's a recommended equipment list in the book bonuses:

http://bit.ly/TE-bookbonuses

You don't have to go and stand under the shower all the time. It can be nice when you have a shower, but heat needs to be done frequently throughout the day.

I used to say heat three times a day, but I had a couple of clients recently heal faster and better by using the heat more frequently. Now I recommend this as the gold standard; if you can heat every hour, heat every hour, and it's for 10 minutes, particularly the neck because it is often involved. The upper traps, the stress muscles are often involved, get heat on there too. We need to relax those off. The forearm is often very tight because the body recognizes there's an injury to the elbow and it wants to take the stress and strain away from that area. That stress and strain is going to go elsewhere and can make those tissues tight too. If those tissues stay tight, you will not achieve full, complete healing. So, we need to relax those tissues off and heat does that very nicely.

The heating pads I particularly like are generally the ones that go in the microwave. They tend to mold around the area a little better than the plug-in ones. The electric ones don't tend to be as malleable. The microwave ones also have a bit of weight to them because they have beads, seeds or corn inside them, and that gentle pressure on the tissues can also help for relaxation.

If you already have a heating pad or a hot water bottle, go and get it right now. Put it in the microwave for a couple of minutes and then come back. Go on, go and do it. Right now, go on. It's going to help.

When you are heating, you are going to heat your neck. You are going to heat your upper traps. You're going to heat your shoulder. You're going to heat your forearm and elbow, unless it is acute, if you feel you've irritated that elbow, you will ice the elbow instead.

Make sure that you are comfortable when you heat. If you're not, change it, we don't want to affect the skin. I have seen people who have used heat that is too hot for them and they got a discoloration of the skin. That is not okay. When I say discoloration, I don't just mean redness. That's normal. It's a more permanent discoloration which does not fade after a few minutes, like the redness would. It stays for a few weeks, and that is damage to the skin and we don't want that. So, when you are putting the heat on, I want you to be feeling a comfortable warmth, that feels relaxing.

If you get too hot your muscles will tense up. That is not what we're trying to achieve. We are trying to get relaxation of the tissues, not tightening them up. The tensing is what pulls on the tendon and makes it hurt. The relaxation is going to relieve tension in the muscle and, therefore, on the tendon and allow it to heal.

Ice, Ice, Baby

You do not need a gigantic ice pad for this. I have little round ones in my clinic, and I give them to my tennis elbow clients.

A tiny little ice pack that you can just get right on that irritated area is immensely helpful. A packet of frozen peas can work as well as anything. Just don't eat the peas afterwards because when they've been on your elbow, they will thaw and then you're going to refreeze them. Just put a little packet of frozen peas into a Ziploc bag, just in case it splits, and you can use that on your elbow.

Now, if you are not in an acute phase, as in it's not really early in your journey. You've had this for a while, it's been irritating you for a few weeks or months, then you can get heat on the elbow. Remember that I said the tendon does not have a very good blood supply, so we want to increase the blood flow around that area? We want to increase the blood supply to the tendon as much as we can naturally, and heat will do that beautifully.

If you think about when you put a heating pad on, and when you take it off, the skin is pink underneath. You've got the circulation going. The same can be said for ice. If you put an ice pack on your elbow and leave it on there for 5 to 10 minutes before you take it off, the skin is going to be pink underneath. You've got the circulation going, but ice tends to then constrict the blood vessels. You're not going to get quite the same effect as with the heat, which is why we use heat and ice for different reasons.

We use ice to help with swelling because it constricts the vessels. Heat opens everything up, and you get a big influx of blood into the area. That's the reason we don't use heat in the acute phase because we don't want a big rush of blood to an area that is very recently injured. It's already bleeding. If we put heat on and get extra blood flow into the area it will make it worse. Therefore, for the first three days of any new injury, ice only. After the first three days, you can choose. Most of my clients prefer heat. Every now and again, somebody will prefer ice. That's okay. It's a personal choice, but just know that heat will get the blood flow going just a little better than the ice will. However, if ice is helpful for you for numbing the pain, use it.

When you're using ice, you need to make sure you are protecting the skin. You've got your packet of frozen peas out of the freezer and to protect the skin you can either wrap a damp towel, a kitchen towel, or a tea towel around the frozen peas before you put them onto your elbow. We do not want the frozen peas or the ice pack sticking to your skin because when you take it off, your skin can become damaged. You'll rip the top layer of your skin off and then we won't be able to ice or heat it until it has healed. Don't slow your healing down.

It's essential that if you are putting ice on to your elbow to wrap it in a damp towel first. I will even go so far as to say, just to be doubly sure it's not going to stick, use a very thin layer of oil on the skin. Then with the damp towel on the elbow, that's going to protect the skin for sure. It can be any kind of oil. It doesn't have to be anything special. I've had clients who have used vegetable oil or olive oil that they had in the kitchen. If you want to use a vitamin E oil, that's entirely up to you, but do not go out and buy anything special. You don't need to. What you've got in your kitchen cupboard right now is quite sufficient. Just use the thin layer of oil and wrap it with the damp towel, get the ice on there for 10 minutes maximum. If it becomes uncomfortable, take it off. Any strategy you use, needs to be completely pain free. If it's not, something's wrong and we need to change it.

Posture Rules

"If you did nothing else, but improved your posture, you would feel so much better." I hear myself saying these words a lot because it's true. We spend so much time and energy trying to figure out which exercise you need to do, or which supplement to take, or which doctor is the best one to see, when in fact, if we just sat a little straighter or stood a little taller and kept our spine in neutral when we're in bed, we maybe wouldn't have to focus so much on the other things.

Sitting puts a lot of stress and strain on the spine. Which puts a lot of stress and strain on the nerves and the other soft tissues. Tendons and nerves are very closely correlated. If you have a tendon problem such as tennis elbow, you are 86% likely to have some kind of nerve issue too [27.] More on this later.

Posture-wise, we are designed to have that little curve in our lower back (see the first photo). That's called the lumbar lordosis.

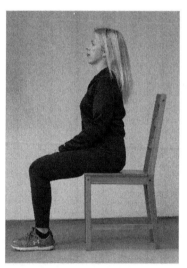 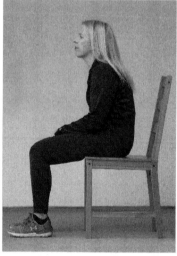

Sitting in poor posture is going to make your healing process last longer. This is because when the spine is in a poor position, the soft tissues around it, including nerves, can be irritated.

Being in a good posture with your earlobe, shoulder and hips in a nice straight line (if you're looking side on), is going to be helpful in reducing your healing time.

When you are sitting in a chair, move your hips all the way to the back of the chair and use the backrest, making sure you've got something supporting your lumbar lordosis, the little curve in your lower back. If you have a chair that has a lumbar support, that little curved support for your low back, use it by just resting back against it. If your chair doesn't have a lumbar support, if it's a flat backed chair, you can roll up a towel and use it in that space. If you are out and about, you can roll up your sweater or roll up your jacket and use it as a support.

We're supposed to have that little curve in our lower back, that S shape through our spine. That's why modern car seats have the lumbar support that supports your lower back. If you're sitting in an ergonomic desk chair, it has that little lumbar support too. You can absolutely recreate this with pillows, cushions or a rolled-up towel.

You've probably got a lumbar support in your car that you can tweak to fit you and be comfortable. If it's there, use it. It may even be similar in your office chair. If you've got a great office chair at home, brilliant. If you're like a lot of people, you may be sitting on a dining room chair or a kitchen chair. That's not ideal but utilize a small cushion or a rolled-up towel to transform it into an ergonomic seat that your body will appreciate.

Sitting in good posture, having your lumbar lordosis supported, is where the spine is designed to be. It's where there's the least amount of abnormal stress and strain going through the spine, and that's where we want to try and keep it. Sitting puts the most stress and strain on our back. You're actually better off standing up rather than sitting. If you have an irritated nerve associated

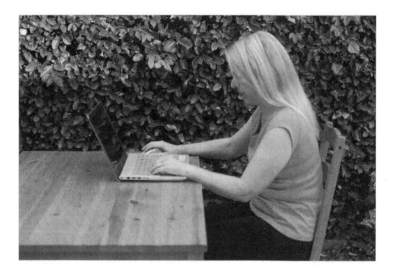

with your tennis elbow, you can often feel the nerve symptoms more when you are sitting at your desk. If you get a tingling, pins and needles or a numbness sensation, you may well move and you settle it down. However, then you go back to sitting in that position, and guess what? It's going to keep coming back.

So, your challenge for today is to be sitting in better posture. I challenge you to set the timer on your phone for 20 minutes so that when the timer goes off, you stand up, sit back down in good posture and reset your timer. What happens when we are sitting and working on our laptops, watching TV, or surfing the internet, you will get sucked into that activity, and before you know it, all your good intentions are going to be gone because the screen just sucks you in. That's the reason for setting your timer for 20 minutes because, after 20 minutes, you're probably down in that C-shaped curve. You need a little reminder. If you don't have a little external reminder like your phone, you're going to end up getting an internal reminder, which will be pain, and we don't want to get to that point.

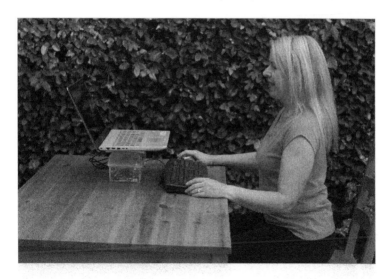

Set your timer for 20 minutes, stand up, sit back down, good posture, reset your timer, and carry on doing whatever it was you're doing. This strategy does not take you away from your desk. If you're working from home, it doesn't take you away from your work. It just breaks up the day. This can be transformational. I have had a number of clients who have literally just done this one strategy and it makes such a difference to how they're feeling, So, please try it. I want you to try it. Give it a go. See how it feels and see how easy it is. It's not going to take any time out of your day. You literally stand up and sit down. It's less than a second. But if you do it consistently through the day, for every 20 minutes while you're sitting, you will notice a difference.

I am going to answer one question that I get asked all the time. "Well, can I not just wear one of those devices that holds me in a good posture?" That's a really good question. The answer is yes, you could, but when you put something external like that on, it may pull you and force you into a good position. Then the tissues underneath, that is the muscles, will realize that something else is doing its job and those muscles will switch off. As a result, if you wear a back support or one of the posture devices that go around your shoulders and pull your shoulders back to try and keep you upright, anything external like that will cause a weakening of the muscles and we don't want that because then you become completely reliant on that device, whatever it is.

Our spine is designed to have curves. These curves allow our spine to move in the way that it is designed to and also to absorb stress and strain in the most effective way. If those curves flatten out, the spine is less effective at absorbing strain and tissues may become damaged. This is where the term "Neutral spine" comes in. What we mean by "Neutral spine" is the naturally occurring position where there is the least amount of abnormal stress or strain on the spine.

Let's find your "Neutral Spine" position right now. If you are sitting reading this book, focus in on the position that you are currently sitting in. How does your spine feel? Is it comfortable? If not, why not?

Arch your back as much as you can comfortably, then round it into the opposite direction as much as you comfortably can. Go from one extreme of the movement to the other extreme of the movement a few times. Make a mental note of how it feels when you are at the end of each motion. Now stop yourself in the middle. Feel how there's less stress and strain on your spine now? Welcome to neutral.

We just discovered that "Neutral Spine" is where the least amount of abnormal stress and strain goes through the spine. What position does sitting tend to put us in? Have a quick check right now, are you sitting in neutral? I'd love it if you were. It's highly likely you're sitting in somewhat of a flexed position. That is a rounded "C" shaped curve of the spine. We learned above that any position outside of neutral, puts more stress through the spine. While this is not always a bad thing, for example you need to be able to bend over to feed the dog, that's normal movement of the spine, but, when we stay in that position for long periods of time, that's when problems can occur.

If we were to stay in the flexed "C" shaped curve for a while, there would start to become some changes within the tissues. The muscles on the back side of the spine would be stretched out. Not too much of a problem initially, but over time, stretched out muscles are unable to function properly, as they have less tissue to get hold of to switch on. If muscles can't switch on properly, they start to weaken. Uh-oh. Weaker muscles? Doesn't sound like a good thing, right? This is the reason my program includes strengthening exercises from the spine to the tips of the fingers and everything in between. We want to make sure that there are no weaknesses or muscle imbalances that could cause symptoms to return.

Relative Rest

Relative rest means avoiding anything that makes it hurt. You're not taking to your bed or putting your arm in a sling, but you are avoiding things that irritate it. Sometimes, this is easier said than done if the irritating factor is your job. However, there may well be things in your day that you don't actually have to do. You might want to do them but ask yourself if you really have to do them.

For example, I had a client who irritated her elbow by cleaning her baseboards. When I asked her why she was doing this irritating activity, she replied that they were dirty and needed cleaning before her family came over for dinner. This is not an essential activity. She *wanted* her baseboards to be clean, but they really didn't *need* to be done. I'll bet her family didn't even notice her baseboards, but they sure noticed her wincing in pain when she reached for her wine glass. Get my drift? There are certain activities that we can choose to do, or not.

Ergonomics

Many people ask, "What's the best office chair or the best mouse?" or similar questions, and the answer is "It depends." We're all different, and what's right for one person isn't necessarily going to be remotely right for another. The best advice I can give anyone is "Go and try them out."

You need to find a chair that is supportive, ideally with a high back rest that extends all the way up to allow your head to rest on it. Think of the supportive seat with a headrest in your car. A lumbar support is very helpful but can be added as an external cushion. Your feet should rest comfortably on the floor, if you're a little on the short side, like me, using a footrest is essential to stop you from dangling.

How about sitting on a ball? Try it and see. Some people really like it and are comfortable. Some people are not. How about the chair that you sit on with support going through your knees? How are your knees? The right chair is essential if you do spend a lot of time sitting at a desk.

Standing desks can be a great option for people who work at a desk all day. They give you the option to change your position and avoid the poor position of sitting all day. It's important to be able to vary the position, as most people are not comfortable to be standing in one position all day either.

If you are sitting in the car, make sure you are using all the support, and resting your head back on the headrest. Office chairs always used to be really low. They would just come up to shoulder blade level and your head was left free. Many office chairs now have that additional head support, which is brilliant. If you have one of those chairs, use it. Make sure you are nice and upright. Use the chair and then scoot yourself underneath the desk so that you can be in a nice straight position. In addition, make sure that the monitor is at eye level.

If you work on a laptop, you have to look down. If you are going to sit for eight hours a day because you're working from home on the laptop, that's going to be a problem for your posture. What I advise clients to do is to take their laptop, raise it up and use it as their monitor. Then, it's at eye level. Have a separate keyboard and mouse down below, and then you can work on a laptop perfectly well in beautiful posture.

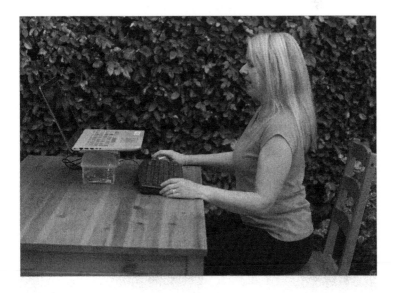

Braces

You don't need to rush out and buy fancy braces. There are all kinds of braces out there for tennis elbow. The classic one is the strap that goes around your forearm. Most people don't know how to use those correctly and they put them right over the area that hurts. It's supposed to go underneath the sore spot, on the muscles, and it goes on as tightly as you can have it without your hand going blue or tingling. That's how it takes the pressure off the tendon.

Do I recommend these all the time? No, I don't. The reason is similar to my answer regarding posture devices. Once you put an external brace on, the muscles underneath switch off because they recognize that something else is doing their job. They don't need to do the work, so they switch off. Part of the problem in tennis elbow is a weakening of the muscles and if you put a brace on, that's going to happen faster, and it is going to be more pronounced. For that reason, you're going to get more weakness faster with the brace on.

There are times when I will suggest people use them. If a client is moving to a new house, they're going to be packing boxes, and they're going to be lifting. Stressing the tendon is going to be unavoidable. The gold standard is to have somebody else do all the lifting and moving. But if you can't and you know you're going to have to do it and it's unavoidable, the brace can be helpful to take the pressure off the tendon.

I had a client who was a sushi chef, it was just before Christmas and he couldn't take any time off. He wore a brace because he had to work at the time. There are certain circumstances where I will say wear it because it will help to protect the tendon, but it is not a long-term fix. If you can change your activities so you don't have to wear the brace, that is much more preferable.

Sleep

A lot of clients will tell me they cannot sleep at night as their elbow really bothers them. Sleep is essential for healing. We heal when we are asleep. Try and get eight hours of sleep if you can.

I know it's really hard, especially if you've got kids or you have to get up early for work. Something I have found really helpful recently has been using an eye mask and earplugs. Something simple like that. They block out light and sound and I sleep much better.

If you can get a good night's sleep, you are going to heal better and faster. There are many things you can do, such as changing your pillow if it's uncomfortable. Simple things like not having caffeine before you go to bed can help. Cutting down on screen time just before you go to bed can also make a huge difference because the blue light from the screens wakes our brains up. Once the sun's gone down, we should be limiting our screen time. We need to limit the blue light from screens, so we allow our brains to go to sleep.

We should also try to stick to a bedtime routine. Like we have for kids when they are little, it's upstairs, bath, PJs, story, bed. Their little bodies get used to that routine. Well, our big bodies would like routine as well. We are creatures of habit. Try and stick to the same time going to bed every night and try and stick to the same time waking up every morning. Don't shift it just because it's the weekend or a holiday but try and stick to the same routine. You're going to find you will get a better quality of sleep. If you get a better quality of sleep, you're going to feel better and heal faster.

Some people adopt the fetal position in bed. Tennis elbows don't tend to like this very much. When we're lying in bed, we are still for eight hours, or however long we're asleep and our circulation slows down. Remember we want to get that circulation going. We want that influx of blood to the area because the blood brings the building blocks for healing that the tendon needs. The circulation slows down when we're in bed and that can increase the irritation in that area. It tends to be more comfortable in a straight position. There are soft braces on the market that can be helpful in this situation. You can also just use a towel, rolled into a sausage shape, and put it along your arm and then hold it in place by gently wrapping a bandage around it, something that is stretchy, not tight, but just to hold it in place so that it can bend, but can't bend all the way up.

The right mattress and pillow can also be immensely helpful. But which is the best? This is another question I get asked a lot. Unfortunately, there is no gold standard when it comes to mattress choice or pillow selection. I love a memory foam mattress, but many people don't. What I suggest is to head to the mattress store and take a good book with you. When you find a mattress that you think will work for you, settle yourself down onto it and read your book for 20 minutes. Ignore the salesperson for that time and just relax. How do you feel at the end of the 20 minutes? If you feel any kind of aches and pains, that's not the mattress (or pillow) for you. But, if you feel great at the end of the 20 minutes, that's the one for you.

Pills, Potions And Lotions

Pain medications can help if you've been prescribed them and you need to take them. Let's go back to the person who can't sleep because the elbow's very painful. If you cannot sleep, you cannot heal. Our bodies heal when we're asleep. If you need to take a pain medication before you go to bed to get a good night's sleep, that's ok to do because you need to sleep well so that you can start healing. If you're not sleeping, you're not going to be healing.

Anti-inflammatories or muscle relaxers would be similar. If you need to use them to be comfortable to sleep, take them, if they've been prescribed to you. Obviously, ask your doctor about these. However, if you've been prescribed them and you need them, take them. On the other hand, if you're taking a medication and it seems to make no difference to you, ask your doctor about it.

Many people try creams or topicals, which you rub onto the area. An anti-inflammatory cream or gel can be helpful in that very early acute phase. If you have an "itis" it can be helpful. I think sometimes the massaging, the actual moving of the soft tissues is what can be helpful too. It's going to increase the circulation to the area, and we know that is helpful.

Lots of clients ask me about Cannabidiol or CBD. It is not my area of expertise. However, I will pass on the information that a lot of my clients find relief when using it. There are so many different types of CBD. I suggest you talk to your doctor and see if they recommend any one in particular. There are different ways of using CBD, as a tincture, which is a little oil droplet that you take. There are edibles, which can be gummies and there's the topical which you put on, just like the anti-inflammatory gel. If you are interested to try one of these options, ask your doctor for a recommendation.

Nutrition

I mentioned earlier that the circulation brings the building blocks for healing in the bloodstream. Those building blocks for healing need to come from the nutrition; the food, the drink, the supplements we take in. Now, to heal a tendon, you need protein. Protein is what makes up that tendon and protein is needed to heal it [28.] If you are not getting enough protein in your diet, your body will take it from somewhere else. It knows it needs protein and it will take it from your source of protein in your body, which is your muscles.

If you eat a good balanced diet, you don't have to take any supplements. If you want to take them, that's completely fine. There is nothing on the market right now that will boost tendon healing, but a good healthy, balanced diet, making sure you're getting enough protein, making sure you're getting enough calcium, making sure you're getting enough of all of the nutrients that you need for healing and for being healthy is going to be beneficial in your healing journey. I recommend a Mediterranean diet as a good go to. You can find information about how to incorporate a Mediterranean diet into your life on many healthy lifestyle websites.

One supplement I have started to recommend recently is Lions Mane. Lions Mane is a supplement derived from the Lions Mane mushroom and is marketed as a memory enhancer or brain booster. I first heard about this supplement a couple of years ago, when I was working with a client who had had a severe injury to his shoulder causing nerve damage to his arm. He was a yoga instructor and as such was very keen on natural remedies. He made the fastest recovery from a nerve injury that I have ever seen, and he put it down to his taking Lions Mane.

Since working with him, and witnessing the amazing recovery he made, I have recommended this supplement to clients who describe nerve symptoms. This may be tingling, pins and needles, numbness or pain, that I recognize as being nerve in origin, and they all seem to benefit from taking Lions Mane. If you are unsure whether this would be a good choice for you, ask your doctor about it.

Another supplement that a number of clients have found useful is magnesium. These particular clients were struggling with increased muscle tension or cramping. They found great relief by taking a supplement of magnesium. My husband swears by an Epsom salts bath after a long bike ride or run. Ask your doctor if this could be helpful for you.

Hydration

In conjunction with nutrition, we need to consider hydration. One of the major causes of pain in tennis elbow is excessive tension in the forearm muscles, which then pulls on the injured tendon. If we are dehydrated, this can make muscle tension worse. A healthy goal is to drink 8 glasses of water per day. The side effect of this will be less muscle tension, which is a great side effect to have.

When considering hydration, it's important to know that certain drinks can lead to dehydration and an increase in muscle tension. Drinks in this category would include highly caffeinated drinks such as strong coffee, colas and energy drinks. Alcohol is also a cause of dehydration. When we are trying to heal a tendon, look at whether you need to make small changes in your nutrition and hydration.

Cardio Exercise

We just learned that our body is not designed to be in a sitting position all day, so what is it designed for? Think back 10,000 years or so; anyone remember back that far? There were no chairs, no phones, no laptops, no tablets. We were running around the fields, looking for food, chasing animals, and picking berries. They are not designed to be sitting all day in a concrete box or sitting all day in a metal box. It was not designed to be chair shaped. It was designed to be out there running and exploring. You get the picture? That's truly what this body of ours is designed for. So, movement is essential for its wellbeing.

Good nutrition, adequate sleep, proper hydration and being outside and seeing green things, are all essential for our body to work most efficiently and effectively.

I'm sure you've already heard about most of the things I mentioned above, but what about the "being outside and seeing green things" part? This is a hugely underutilized strategy that is essential for our body's wellbeing. If someone has been experiencing pain for longer than 3 months, they have chronic pain. By definition, discomfort that lasts longer than 3 months is defined as being chronic. We are learning more about chronic pain all the time. One of the things that we have learned is that chronic pain produces biochemical and anatomical changes in the brain [25]. These changes can be reversed by "Rebooting" the brain [29.] Getting out into nature can do this. This is why I advise all my clients to do 30 minutes of cardio exercise every day, preferably outside, so that they can see green things like plants, trees, flowers and grass.

The reason I want you to get outside to do your cardio exercise is I want you to see green things. It gets a little bit woo-woo, but if you see green things, if you see nature, that is the way we can reboot the brain. Right now, if you have chronic pain, your nervous system is screaming at your brain and you are in a cycle of chronic pain. We have to break that cycle. The way we break that cycle is by getting back into nature. By rebooting the brain, we calm the nervous system down. The nervous system is going to stop sending all of those pain messages and you can start your healing journey. If we don't do that, you're going to struggle to heal.

Now there are different forms of exercise. What I'd like you to start today is cardio exercise. "But Emma it's my elbow. I'm not going to run around on my hands." No, you're not. But you are going to do cardio exercise. Reason being, you need to increase your circulation. You need your blood whizzing around your body. You need to get an increase in blood flow to your tendon. A really good way of whizzing your circulation round is cardio exercise. That can be as simple as walking and that's what I'm going to ask you to do today. I want you to do one minute of walking today. That's it. One minute. It's super simple. Nobody can say "I don't have time to go." It's one minute. You literally step out of the door and start your timer. Walk 30 seconds. Turn around and walk back. Done. Achieved. Check it off the list because just doing cardio exercise is going to increase your circulation.

Are you going to stick with one minute every day? No, you're going to build up slowly. But we will build you up every single day, no days off. The cardio exercise that you're going to be doing is for rehab. You're doing the cardio exercise for your tendon, that is, to get your circulation going and whizzing around so that your tendon can heal. You need to do the cardio exercise every single day and you will increase the duration by a minute each day. So, tomorrow you're going to do two minutes, the day after, three minutes, the day after, four minutes, so that you're slowly over time increasing it until you get to 30 minutes.

I want you to be able to do cardio exercise for half an hour. It will take you a month from today to get there, which is why you're starting today because if you start next week, it's going to be a month from then. Start today, one minute of cardio exercise, that's all I'm recommending you do. It's super easy. If you are used to exercising, start 30 minutes of cardio exercise today, preferably outside. If you live somewhere that is very hot, choose your time of day. Go first thing in the morning, or go last thing at night, if that feels better for you. Maybe don't go out in the heat of the middle of the day. If you live somewhere that is very wet, maybe don't go out in the rain. Maybe walk around the house instead. If you want to get out there with your umbrella, go for it. Just don't slip, be sensible. If you live somewhere that is very cold, choose your time and choose your place.

I've developed a month-long Cardio Challenge that I implement in my Facebook group, to take you from zero to 30 minutes of cardio every day. If you'd like to join the next one, join my group here:

www.facebook.com/groups/tenniselbowrelief

You can download my Cardio Calendar here:

http://bit.ly/TE-bookbonuses

Mental Cardio
Heart Health vs Brain Health

We are now learning that these 2 factors are intricately intertwined. You won't have one without the other. Take the cardio exercise we just learned about. Before today, you probably just associated cardio exercise with physical fitness, but cardio exercise plays a huge role in mental fitness too. It makes sense really when you consider the increase in circulation we get with cardio exercise. You get an increase in blood flow to the muscles and tendons. But you also get that increase in circulation to the brain. Add on to that the images of nature that we talked about. This can "reboot" the brain out of its chronic pain cycle.

There are other strategies I advocate regarding the mind-body connection. Here they are and reasons why each one is important. You may feel that these are so similar that you just choose to do one. However, you would be missing out on the distinct and important benefits each one brings to the healing of tennis elbow. I encourage you to add them all to allow you to heal in the fastest time possible.

Relaxation

We talked about the muscles being tight. The muscles are going to be tight in your forearm, in your neck, in your upper traps and around the shoulder. We need to relax them off. Progressive relaxation is something that you can utilize to do that.

Progressive relaxation is something that I have taught for a long time. Now with the wonders of YouTube, you can find progressive relaxation on the web. Go to YouTube and type in progressive relaxation and about 2 million different options will come up. They are essentially guided relaxations that you can listen to. That's what I want you to do. You're going to listen to them and find one that you like. It might be the way that the speaker sounds that resonates with you. It might be the tone of their voice. It might be that you like a British accent. It might be that you don't. It might be that they have the sound of waves crashing in the background. (That would be my favorite.) It might be that there's rain, or a waterfall or water trickling or classical music or whale song. There are so many different types, but you need to find what's right for you. Download it onto your phone or your iPad, get into bed at night, click it on. Go through the progressive relaxation, fall asleep and sleep like a baby. Remember we talked about bedtime routine before. This is perfect for that bedtime routine.

Well, what is progressive relaxation? It's progressive, we start at the top and work our way down. Or you can start from the toes and work your way up, but the goal is to get relaxation of all the different muscle groups. I tend to start from my toes and work my way up. I say, I tend to, because I use this strategy myself. If ever I go to bed and I can't fall asleep, I use progressive relaxation to help relax my body and allow me to get to sleep. So, I suggest that you do this at nighttime when you get into bed. If you fall asleep before you've finished, perfect. You don't get more relaxed than that.

This is how I go through my progressive relaxation:

- I start from the tips of my toes and I work my way up. What I want you to do is lie on your back, get into a comfortable position, and close your eyes. Start with your toes. Curl your toes as tightly as you can and hold the contraction tight, tight, tight, tight, tight, holding it for 10 seconds. Then you release and literally just relax.

- Then you pull your toes back towards you as far as you can, hold them tight, tight, tight, tight, tight, tight, tight release.

- Then you're going to move on to the ankles. You're going to point your feet down, as far as they can go. Hold it tight, tight, tight, tight, tight, for 10 seconds, then release.

- Now pull your feet back and you hold it tight, tight, tight, tight, tight, tight, tight, for 10 seconds and release.

- Then you're going to push your knees down. So, you push your knees as straight as they'll go. Tight, tight, tight, tight, tight, tight, tight, really tighten all those muscles and drop. It's just a release. It's a drop.

- Squeeze your glutes, your butt muscles (bum if you're in the UK). 10 second hold. Release.

- Pull the tummy muscles in. Suck that tummy in as much as you can pull, pull, pull, pull, pull, pull, pull, pull, relax.

- You're going to pull your shoulders back to the bed. So, you're going to press them back behind you. Squeeze, squeeze, squeeze, squeeze, release.

- Now, depending on how your arm feels, you can either do the arm exercises or not. So, if you are going to do them, you're going to straighten your elbows out as much as you can. Generally, that's okay for most people. If it's not okay for you, don't do it. But you press your elbows as straight as you can. Press, press, press, press, press, press, press 10 seconds and release.

- And then you're going to make tight fists. If that is not okay for you, don't do it. 10 second hold, then release.

- Spread the fingers out wide. We're going to hold that for 10 seconds. Squeeze, squeeze, squeeze, release.

- Now we're going to take the shoulders up towards the ears. Tight, tight, tight, tight, tight, tight, tight, tight, tight. Release.

- You're going to press your head back into the pillow. Press, press, press, press, press, press, press, press, release.

- Now we get to the face ones and these are my favorite. So, you're going to screw your face up into a frown as tightly as you can, like really tight, tight, tight, release,

- Then a big wide smile, tight, tight, tight, tight, tight, tight, tight, relax, and then just drop and rest.

- You will literally feel your body just sinking and melting into the bed. It feels fantastic to do that.

Well done! That's your first progressive relaxation session completed.

You can find this in video format in the book bonuses here:

http://bit.ly/TE-bookbonuses

Basically. the theory behind progressive relaxation is that when you do a maximum contraction of a muscle, it is followed by maximum relaxation of the same muscle. That's the way the muscles work and we're using that strategy for progressive relaxation. We're going to get the full relaxation of the muscle as we do that. As I say, it all needs to be comfortable. If it's not comfortable in any way, don't do it and move on to do a different body part. That's fine. I start from my toes and work my way up. That's just easier for me. If you want to start from the top of your head and work your way down, that's completely fine. If you fall asleep before you finish, brilliant, you are nice and relaxed. Sometimes you might need to go through it two or three times, and that's ok.

This is something else you're going to start today. You're going to do this tonight. When you get into bed, you're going to go through your progressive relaxation. You don't have to listen to a video. You can just go through it in your head. That's what I do. I don't listen to anything. I go through it in my head. The listening to something can be nice to really cue you into what you should be feeling as you learn this new technique. It's training you how to do it. You're going to start progressive relaxation tonight when you get into bed.

Meditation

Meditation is something that is becoming more mainstream. I always used to think it was a little bit woo woo, and it wasn't really my thing, but the more I learn about it, the more we all should be doing this. It is so good for our brains. It's so good for the brain chemistry.

The reason I advise my clients to meditate is twofold. One, it really helps with relaxation and the body awareness of this relaxation. You become aware of tension and you can feel the relaxation. That's the physical aspect of it. The other side of it is you are resting your brain. This is crucial for chronic pain sufferers to break the cycle of their pain. Chronic pain is pain that someone's been feeling for three months or longer. If you've had tennis elbow for longer than three months, you have chronic pain. Anything less than three months is acute or subacute. It is not chronic. By three months or more and you are experiencing chronic pain.

If you go back 20 years ago, we did not know very much about chronic pain. We were really just starting to learn about it and truly we are still learning about it now. New research is coming out all the time. What we have learned about chronic pain is that it changes the biochemistry in your brain and it actually changes the anatomy of your brain. The reason being is that the nervous system is sending pain messages to the brain. The nervous system is sending pain, pain, pain, pain, and the brain is essentially saying okay, what should I do about it? That's been going on and on and on and on. This process changes the chemicals in your brain, and it changes the anatomy of your brain. However, these changes are reversible. Meditation helps to relax the brain and allows that changing back of the biochemistry in the brain [30.]

You need to start doing meditation, so that we are giving the brain a rest, and calming down the nervous system. Now for learning meditation, there are some fantastic, guided meditations available. There are apps; Calm is an app that you can use for guided meditation. Headspace is another one. At the time of writing, both of them have free versions as well as some paid content too. You can access guided meditation on YouTube. I really love Deepak Chopra. You can find him on YouTube and Facebook. Therefore, meditation is something that I challenge you to do. I challenge you to start meditation today for the reasons that I mentioned above, just 5 minutes will help.

Visualization

The last thing I'm going to talk about is visualization. I know it sounds similar, meditation and visualization, but they work in very different ways. In meditation, we are giving the brain a rest. We're not thinking about anything. In visualization, we're using our imagination. We're really using our brain to visualize things in intense detail. Athletes use visualization often through their training. Research has actually shown that strength can be gained by visualization alone [31.]

I was actually introduced to visualization as a gymnast, back in my younger days. I can remember our coach got us all to think about a teacup. At the time we would snigger to each other. What the heck is he going on about? Think of a teacup! But that is how he would start our visualization sessions. Then we would visualize ourselves going through the gymnastic moves that we were learning. You immerse yourself in the experience and imagine yourself performing the movement flawlessly, over and over again.

I use this strategy for all my sports clients. I have a number of elite athletes that I work with, though anybody who plays any sport, from weekend warriors to the occasional tennis player, can use visualization. It is effective even for people who are not sports people. I work with a lot of musicians and they use visualization of playing their instruments. It works even for people who just have one particular task that they want to be able to accomplish, pain-free. Maybe it's picking up a bottle of water, picking up your cup of coffee, or picking up a gallon of milk. We can use visualization to help achieve it.

Visualization is an incredibly powerful tool for working on the brain. It kind of tricks the brain a little bit. You're not tricking it in a bad way, but we're tricking it into thinking that your body can do that particular activity pain-free. For example, I had a client who was a softball player, and she couldn't play because her elbow was bothering her. She visualized pitching every day. She visualized throwing every day. She visualized batting every day and in intense detail. You've got to use all of your senses with visualization. You've got to see it. You've got to hear it. You've got to smell it. You've got to touch it. You've got to taste it. You've got to be totally in that moment.

We're going to start doing visualization today as well. You can do this anywhere. Ideally, you want to be somewhere quiet. You're not going to do this when you're driving around in a car or are in a busy work area or you have kids screaming in the background, although I can tune my kids out really well. You want to be in a quiet place so you can really focus on what you're doing. You can do it lying down, or sitting, if that's more comfortable. Close your eyes, so that you are immersing yourself in the moment.

Let's think back, to the softball player who's going to visualize throwing. She is going to feel the ball in her hand. She's going to feel where her arm is, though, she's not moving. She's resting in the same position, but she is feeling it as though she is there. She feels the sun on her face. She takes a step forward and she cocks her arm back and then she throws the ball and she throws it perfectly. The thing about visualization is you are not moving whilst you're visualizing. This is not going to be detrimental at all to your elbow, as you're not doing the motion physically.

What visualization does is it reinforces the neural pathways that your body switches on when you do that particular movement. Let me explain what I mean by that. A neural pathway is basically the message that the brain sends to your muscles to say, switch on, in this way, to perform that task. Now, when you do something so many times, it becomes automatic. Once it's automatic our neural pathways are set. This is motor learning.

Motor learning is best explained by this example I love to use. Imagine a little kid learning to ride a bike because we've all seen them; a young kid on their bike and they're trying to take the training wheels off (stabilizers if you're in the UK). They're trying and trying and they keep falling off and falling off because they haven't got the correct neural pathway set yet. Their brain doesn't know how to send the correct messages. "Which muscles am I switching on to balance and pedal and steer and stay up?" It doesn't know yet. So, they practice, and practice and they fall off, and each time they're getting new information and getting new input. No, that was not right so try a different pathway. No, that was not right. Try a different one.

All of a sudden, they get it and off they go, with the biggest smile on their face and mum and dad running after them. That's motor learning in action. They didn't know how to do a task and all of a sudden, they do. What's happened is they found the correct neural pathway. That is the message that the brain sends down to the muscles and the joints to say, move in this way so you can stay up on that bike and you can keep going.

When they get it, now they're doing it, they are strengthening that neural pathway. They are strengthening it and strengthening it each time they perform the movement. What visualization does is strengthen that neural pathway, without you moving. Your brain will send those messages to the muscles and the joints, to fire in that way, to move in that way. When you make that perfect pitch, when you throw that perfect ball, when you hit that perfect shot, whatever it may be, the brain is going to strengthen those neural pathways.

Right now, you can't play tennis. You can't play golf. You

can't play the drums. You can't play the guitar. You're not lifting. You're not picking your kids up. You're not working out or whatever else you may be prevented from doing. We want to make sure we don't lose the neural pathways associated with those activities, because if we don't use them, we lose them. We don't completely forget how to do the movement, you know you can always ride a bike, but it's probably not as good as if you'd been practicing it the whole time.

We want to keep those neural pathways sharp and strong so that when you are able to get back to hitting that ball, throwing a ball, working out, playing the violin or whatever it is you're going to do, those neural pathways are ready for you to do that activity. That's what visualization will do for you. I challenge you to do visualization today.

Quick Recap

To recap, you've got a lot to try today:

- Heat
- Ice
- Keeping good posture and ergonomics
- Staying pain-free
- Different types of brace (don't do it, if you don't need to)
- Pills or creams (again, don't use them if you don't need them)
- Get a good night's sleep
- Good nutrition and hydration
- Cardio exercise (get out there and get into nature)
- Progressive relaxation
- Meditation
- Visualization.

Do you see how all of these different components, everything that I've taught you, all of them matter? Can you imagine just doing ultrasound on your elbow and not doing the rest of it? It's no wonder people don't get better. If you do all these things, you are going to feel so much better. These strategies are what resolves phase one. Phase one is where you're really feeling the symptoms, where you're really uncomfortable. These self-help strategies will help to get you through this phase. You're on your way to healing.

Check out Chapter 9 for a daily checklist of all the Phase 1 self-help strategies.

This is updated in my Facebook group as new research comes out. Join the Facebook group here:

https://www.facebook.com/groups/tenniselbowrelief

Ready to go from hurt to healed? Find out more about my comprehensive program and all the other bonuses here:

http://bit.ly/TE-bookbonuses

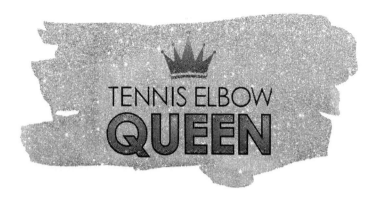

Success Story Snippet

66 She started going out with a friend a few weeks ago to practice softball. She said she is stretching, and her arm feels fine. Thank you so much for taking care of her when everyone else said they couldn't! You are a miracle worker! 99

– CC, Mom of a teenaged female softball player, USA

CHAPTER 7

Phase 2
Normalizing
The Soft Tissues

Getting Soft For The Soft Tissues

Why do we need to stretch? For several reasons, firstly, our muscles accommodate to the stresses and strains put through them. For example, if you spend all day sitting, the muscles and soft tissues at the front of your hips are in a shortened position. Stay there for a prolonged period of time and the soft tissues will shorten. The second reason is that muscle tension or spasm can often be part of the problem. So, what is muscle spasm, and what causes it? Why does it happen?

Muscle spasm, cramp, or Charlie horse, all describe the same thing, a muscle getting so tight that it can't switch itself off or relax. If you've ever experienced this, you know how painful it can be. People need to jump out of bed at night if they get a cramp in the calf muscle. Ouch.

Why does it happen? There are a number of reasons. Firstly, injury, where the body may cause a "splinting" effect to try to protect an injured area. Then the pain you feel can lead to an increase in muscle tension. Hold that injured arm in a poor posture or position, as in our example above when sitting for a long time, and your muscle tension will go up. Conversely, excessive use of the muscle, such as if you've spent two hours pulling weeds, or something similar, can also increase muscle tension.

A hyper-firing nerve is one of the scenarios that doesn't often get addressed. The hyper-firing nerve or hypersensitized nervous system can be a big factor in tennis elbow's stubbornness to heal. This is why many of the strategies I recommend, even in phase 1, address the nervous system. Has it ever been suggested to you to use meditation, progressive relaxation and nature to reboot your brain, in order to heal your elbow? This is what makes my program so different to anything else out there.

Dehydration was mentioned earlier as a situation which can delay healing. It can also increase muscle tension and increase your pain. Occasionally, a lack of salt can also cause problems with normal muscle function, including excessive muscle tension. I discussed supplements that clients have found useful for this issue in the nutrition section earlier.

We Should Learn From The Animals

Every morning when my little dog gets up, he is desperate to come and say "Hi" to me, and his little tail looks like it's going to wag off. However, he doesn't jump out of his bed to come and give me kisses until he has stretched his front legs, and then stretches one of his back legs and then his other back leg. Then and only then, will he come and say "Hi" to his mama. No-one has told animals to stretch when they first get up, they do it instinctively.

Stretches can be very effective as long as you're doing the right ones. Sometimes, you need to stretch in one direction.

Sometimes, you need to stretch in the other direction depending on the cause of the problem. I've had clients tell me, "Well, I tried these exercises on YouTube," because that's what everybody does. They go to Dr. Google, type in their diagnosis and learn about it. Go to YouTube, find the exercises, and do the exercises, but depending on what's causing the issue, you might find the wrong exercises. The wrong exercises are going to make you worse. So, knowing what's causing your problem, points you in the right direction for knowing what's going to heal it.

Stretch it out safely. Stretches should always feel comfortable. They should never illicit, what I call the "Pain Face", you know the one that you pull when you've had a really deep tissue massage, or when you step on a piece of Lego (parents, you feel me?). Stretches should never feel painful. It's ok to feel a stretch sensation, but not pain.

Heat can be really helpful before you stretch too, unless it's within the first three days of a fresh injury in which case you would just use ice. However, a heating pad, a hot shower, a hot towel, any of those things, can be really helpful at increasing circulation to the area. We want to get fresh blood to the area as the blood brings the building blocks for healing that your body needs when it's trying to heal an injury, but heat can also relax off tight muscles. If you've got muscle spasm around the elbow or around the neck and shoulders, that can be uncomfortable in itself. Just think about cramp. If you get cramp in your leg, it's so painful and we want to release that off.

Stretching for flexibility helps to regain range of motion that may have been lost. Sometimes, if we have an injury, we don't want to move that area. If we don't move an area for a while, that area is going to get stiff. This is because our body adapts to the stresses and strains that we put through it. If we're not moving a joint through its full range of motion, the soft tissues around it will shorten to accommodate. While this process in itself is normal, our tissues are accommodating to everything we do, be it marathon training, sitting at a desk all day, or limiting the use of our arm as it's painful, a lack of range of motion is not normal.

Stretching can be a great way to regain the range of motion. Ensure you're holding the stretch comfortably and maintain the stretch statically for 30 seconds. There has been a lot of research done on stretching and its effectiveness and we know that if you hold a stretch for less than 30 seconds, that's a good warm up stretch, but it isn't going to increase your flexibility or your range of motion. However, holding a stretch for at least 30 seconds will lead to an increase in your range and flexibility [32.] 30 seconds will feel like a long time. Time yourself with your watch or your phone, to ensure you are holding it for long enough. If you are able to tolerate holding a stretch for 30 seconds, then you only need to do it once. Repeating it over and over won't gain you any more benefit. However, repeating the stretch little and often throughout the day, preferably after the heat can lead to great increases in healing.

Joints Are Designed To Move

All joints like to move as it's what they are designed to do. Indeed, joints get their nutrition through movement. Joint surfaces are covered with cartilage. The cartilage reduces friction and allows the joint surfaces to move smoothly over each other. When the joints move through their full range of motion, the joint fluid which bathes the joint surfaces, is squeezed out of the cartilage, giving nutrition to the joint. Therefore, if joints don't go through their full range of motion on a regular basis, they get less nutrition, which in turn can lead to the joint becoming stiffer. Joint fluid should be fluidy, which makes sense, right? Although, if joints don't move normally, this fluid can thicken up, a bit like custard, making it harder for the joints to move normally. This also doesn't feel so great. Therefore, you start to move even less, which leads to less nutrition and thicker fluid, which feels bad, So, you move less, and so on and so on and so on. You get the picture? Takes us back to the animals that stretch every time they get out of bed.

My program includes 15 different stretches and soft tissue techniques to work on normalizing the soft tissues in Phase 2. You can learn more about my comprehensive online Tennis Elbow Relief Program in the book bonuses here:

http://bit.ly/TE-bookbonuses

The Best 3 Stretches That We All Should Be Doing

Knee Rolling

This is by far my all-time favorite stretch. If you add this to your daily routine, before you get out of bed each morning, you will start to be able to get out of bed with less stiffness. It works by essentially "oiling the joints", increasing the circulation, stretching out the muscles and soft tissues, even gently moving the nervous system, before you load the spine by getting out of bed. Think about it; you've just spent 8 hours in bed, which is an unloaded position for the body. When we sit up on the edge of the bed, we now have body weight pressing down. Let's warm it up first.

Knee rolling is a super simple exercise that I really like for everybody. I tend to teach people to do this first thing in the morning and last thing at night. Lie down on your back with your knees bent up so your feet are flat on the bed.

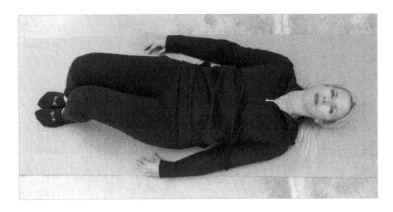

You're just going to let your knees roll from side to side, but your feet don't lift up.

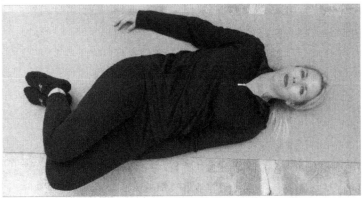

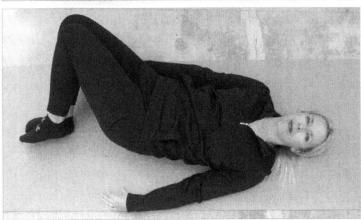

This is not a core exercise. It's not a strengthening exercise. It's a mobility exercise, and you're purely just rolling your knees from side to side. It helps. It moves the joints. It gets the muscles stretching out. It gets the circulation going to the spine area. "But Emma, how is this going to help my elbow?" The reason I use it for my tennis elbow clients is that it mobilizes the nervous system, encouraging good circulation to and within the nervous system and helps to calm it down.

Neck Retractions (a.k.a. Chin Tucks)

This is the first exercise that I give to all my clients. I know it seems weird, as I'm giving you a neck exercise to help you heal your elbow, but it works. For this exercise, you are lying down on your back, so you can do it after you've done the knee rolling. Keep your knees bent up and gently press the back of your head into the pillow. Use just a thin flat pillow, if it feels comfortable. You don't need to hold this position, just get there and then release. Now, remember that all exercises should feel comfortable, so you may need to start with a smaller movement and work up to a full range of motion. That's completely fine. I recommend 10 of these exercises, 3 times per day. You can watch a video of me teaching this exercise and going into the reasons why I use it in the book bonuses:

http://bit.ly/TE-bookbonuses

Upper Traps Stretch

I love this one too. It feels so good. This stretch targets the muscle between the head and the shoulder. These are our stress muscles. 10 minutes in traffic and these tighten up. If you are feeling pain, these tighten up. If they are tight, they can pull on the connective tissue that travels up and over the top of your head causing tension headaches. They can also pull on the neck leading to stiffness. If they pull on the shoulder, that can cause soreness, but it can also squeeze on the nerves, which doesn't help settle the hypersensitivity.

Take the chin down to the chest and then take your ear down to your shoulder. You should feel a stretch in the muscle between the neck and the shoulder. Hold it, comfortably, for 30 seconds. Repeat on the other side. You might find that the affected side is tighter, so stretch it again.

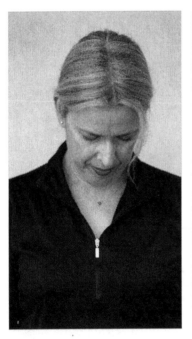 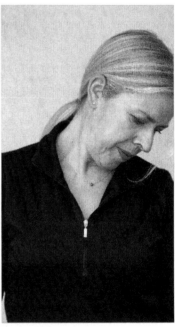

Self-Massage

This is the phase where we use self-massage too. You can use any oil or lotion that you already have around the house, you don't need to go out and buy anything special. Start by gently rubbing around the elbow but avoid the sore spot of the tendon. You can work on the forearm muscles, biceps and triceps muscles of the upper arm too. Even the upper traps, which we just stretched, can benefit from some soft tissue work. The key to this is to keep it comfortable.

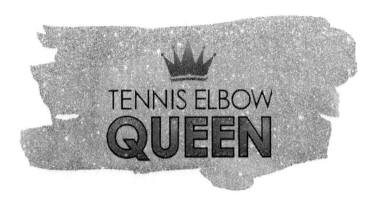

Success Story Snippet

❝ First I wanted to tell you that today's been a pretty good day so I've been really good about not being on the computer or texting on my phone hardly at all!! You are a wealth of information! I've NEVER heard such detailed info! Thank you again for always being available for questions, it means a lot! ❞

— PT, female, 50s, USA

CHAPTER 8

Phase 3
Strengthening

This is where the magic happens.

This has to be my favorite phase of the whole program, as this is where the magic happens, and the tendon heals. I love empowering people to get to and through this phase because I see such a change in their demeanor and outlook once they realise they are in control of their recovery and it can happen.

My program contains 10 specific strengthening exercises which focus on the entire kinetic chain from the core to the fingers and everything in between. If you are aiming to completely resolve your tennis elbow once and for all, you not only need to regain the strength in the weak muscles around the elbow, but also address any weaknesses around the shoulder and spine too. I guide you through these exercises and why it's important to address them.

Here I share the first 3 strengthening exercises for Phase 3. You'll find more for the elbow in the 100-day plan at the back of the book. You can learn more about my complete online Tennis Elbow Relief Program in the book bonuses:

http://bit.ly/TE-bookbonuses

Breathing

Breathing is another essential action our bodies need to stay healthy. There are no flies on me... Right? Keep breathing to stay healthy. Don't stop breathing, that's very unhealthy for your body. I joke, of course. We all know that breathing is a normal part of being alive. If respiration stops, it's not a good situation.

But what about the quality of the breathing? I'm not talking about the quality of the air that you're breathing, although that too is super important. I'm talking about the actual quality of the inhaling and exhaling that you are doing. Have you ever thought about it? Do it now. Just stop reading for a second and take a couple of breaths.

Do you feel the air going deep down into the base of your lungs, or is it staying up at the top of the lungs? Does your tummy fill outwards as you take a deep breath in, dropping gently as you breathe out?

This motion, as automatic as it is, can become less than efficient. If this happens, the breaths tend to become less deep and more shallow. The air at the base of the lungs may become stagnant and as such, how can it promote optimum exchange of oxygen into the body? Poor posture or prolonged sitting are two of the things that can negatively affect good breathing.

You can start practicing good breathing techniques today. Diaphragmatic breathing encourages the optimum use of the diaphragm, which is the major muscle involved in breathing. You can watch me teach this technique in a video in the book bonuses:

http://bit.ly/TE-bookbonuses

Core Of Steel

Ok Emma, stop. Why are we talking about the core, when it's my elbow that hurts? Great question. The simple answer is

"Everything is connected". Let me explain. Many times, when clients have elbow pain, they stop using their elbow, but, then they are not using their arm, so they get weakness there. The muscles around the shoulder blades get weaker. Then the spine and core... You see where I'm going with this. So, when I start a strengthening program, it's all encompassing. Read on.

This is where things get really interesting. Let's talk about everything "Core". I know you've heard the term "Core" and you may even know that it's important to strengthen your core, but how do you do that? Have you checked out some "Core" exercises on Youtube? You may have even tried them. But are they really right for you? Or are you even doing them correctly? It's really helpful to understand a little bit of the background surrounding this elusive structure.

What Is The "Core"?

Simply, the "Core" is a group of muscles that work together to support the spine. Well, that sounds easy enough, right? Let's investigate these muscles one at a time.

Let's start with the abdominals, there are four different sets of abdominal muscles. Three of them are movement muscles, and one of them is a stability muscle. The three that move you are not really your core. It's the one that stabilizes your spine that is the core.

Let's meet the abdominal muscles from the outermost to the most internal.

RECTUS ABDOMINIS a.k.a. YOUR 6-PACK

Yes. It's in there, even if you can't quite see it from the outside. Your 6-pack is essentially your "Sit-up" muscle, as in, if you were to do sit ups, it's your 6-pack muscle that is working. The

4 abdominal muscles are either movement or stability muscles. Rectus Abdominis moves you in the sit up motion, therefore, it is a movement muscle, not a stability muscle. So, your 6-pack is not your core.

OBLIQUUS EXTERNUS ABDOMINIS
a.k.a. EXTERNAL OBLIQUES

Both the internal and external obliques are at the sides of the trunk and control turning of the body. They are movement muscles, not stability muscles.

OBLIQUUS INTERNUS ABDOMINIS
a.k.a. INTERNAL OBLIQUES

As above, both the internal and external obliques are at the sides of the trunk and control turning of the body. Once again, they are movement muscles, not stability muscles.

TRANSVERSUS ABDOMINIS a.k.a. THE CORE

This is the "Core" muscle. Transversus Abdominis is the deepest abdominal muscle, with layers of other muscles and tissue over the top of it. It is a big sheet of muscle, encircling the torso, attaching into the spine and the pelvis. The muscle fibers of Transversus Abdominis are oriented horizontally, so that when they contract, they cause a drawing in or corset type of action to the body. Think back to the olden days when ladies would tighten the ribbons to draw their corset in, that's what Transversus Abdominis does. I like the analogy of Transversus Abdominis being your own inbuilt back brace because that's essentially where it sits and what it does.

So, if you look at the picture, you can color-code it. It's super cool. Color in the rectus abdominis green. This is your six-pack.

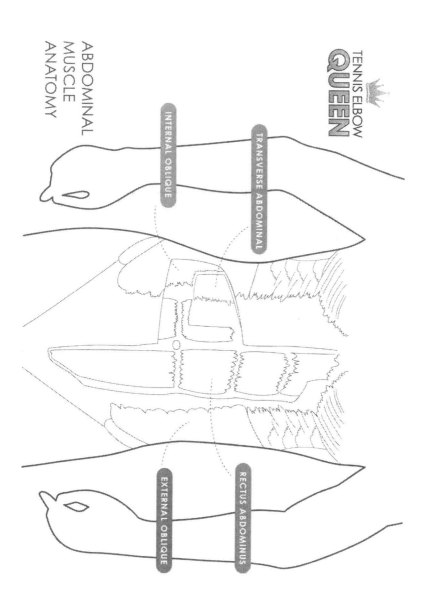

ABDOMINAL
MUSCLE
ANATOMY

TENNIS ELBOW
QUEEN

INTERNAL OBLIQUE

TRANSVERSE ABDOMINAL

EXTERNAL OBLIQUE

RECTUS ABDOMINUS

Next you have the two sets of obliques. Color in the external obliques purple and the internal obliques pink underneath. Then you can see the little holes like little windows going through because essentially, your abdominals are layers of muscle. You've got the two sets of obliques, the internal and the external.

Color the Transversus Abdominis yellow. It is the one that you can see once we've cut through all those different layers of muscle. That's transversus abdominis. That's your core muscle. It is the deepest, the innermost abdominal muscle, supporting you essentially from the belly button and below. It's deep, and there are the layers of the other muscles and different tissues over the top of it before you even get to Transversus Abdominis.

That's the most important core muscle. It's the one that we need to start switching on. People ask me, "Which machine in the gym should I do to work this muscle?" The answer is…there isn't one. There isn't a machine in the gym or an exercise that you can do to just activate it unless you know how to activate it, and that's the challenging part. This muscle can be really lazy.

You have four different sets of abdominals, and the abdominal muscles are really important here. When we talk about the core, we talk about core stability. That helps to take a lot of pressure off the body and to protect the spine.

We just learned that Transversus Abdominis is the "Core" muscle of the abdominals, and great though it is, it doesn't stabilize the spine all by itself. There are 4 muscle groups that work together to form the core. Transversus Abdominis works with the pelvic floor muscles, as both muscles are so internal. They also work with Multifidus, which are tiny little muscles which attach on the spine, from one vertebra to the next. The final muscle that makes up the core is the diaphragm. All 4 of these muscles, Transversus Abdominis, the pelvic floor, Multifidus and the diaphragm, work to stabilize the spine.

Imagine Transversus Abdominis as the corset I described earlier, add in the Multifidus muscles at the back, say, as reinforcement, or boning of the corset. Take the image of those muscles as a cylinder. Now let's add the pelvic floor muscles as the bottom of the cylinder, and the diaphragm as the top, or lid. Now you're thinking about your "Core."

Why Your Core Lets You Down When You Need It Most

There has been a lot of research done on transversus abdominis, including needle EMG studies, which show how and when the muscle activates. This muscle has really been studied quite a lot because, obviously, we know it's super important, and so we've been able to learn lots about it. We know that it switches off if you have back pain [33]. So, the most important muscle that you need to protect your spine, switches off, followed by the little multifidus muscles at the back, and they don't regain strength unless you specifically train it back [34].

Therefore, whenever you have back pain, important muscles have switched off. Other situations that will switch these muscles off as well are pregnancy, because obviously everything gets stretched out through the abdomen when you're pregnant, and depending on how many pregnancies you've had, each time, that muscle is stretched out, it's going to switch off to a degree. Any kind of abdominal injury or surgery will also switch off these muscles. During abdominal surgeries, they're going through these muscles. Pregnancy and C-sections are a double whammy, and if you've had back pain during your pregnancy as well, that's the trifecta right there. Even laparoscopic surgery or keyhole surgery is still going through these muscles and will cause them to switch off, and they don't come back unless you train them back.

If you think about how many of those different scenarios you may have experienced in your life, we've got to wonder, "Is that muscle switching on or not?", because it may not be working for you. A lot of fit and active people, and I would definitely put athletes in that category, can compensate for a weak core by using the other abdominal muscles. It's not normal movement, but it does work. It can be efficient. Whilst you are still working and still training, it can work. A lot of athletes compensate like this.

In my previous sporting life, I worked with a lot of athletes. They could do 400 sit-ups, but they couldn't switch on transversus abdominis. They couldn't activate their core. The muscles on the outside were strong and working so well that they were compensating for it, but then they came to the end of their sporting career, which can be quite a short time span, and they stopped working out as much as they had been doing. They would then start to have issues because the movement abdominal muscles, started to weaken because they just weren't working as much, and transversus abdominis wasn't working for them underneath. We've got to make sure transversus abdominis works correctly and works as it should do.

How Do You Strengthen Your Core?

Isn't this the six-million-dollar question? This is a great question and one that could thoroughly confuse you if you Google it. There are many viewpoints out there on the best exercise to strengthen your core. I've seen many people who have been doing "Core" exercises for a long time, but when we check their

Transversus Abdominis, it's not actually working. How then are they strengthening their core? The answer is, they aren't. They are under the illusion that they are doing core exercises, but as Transversus Abdominis is not switching on, they are not doing what they think they are.

There are some very specific exercises to get this muscle working by itself because as I said, it can be lazy. If your other stomach muscles, any of the other abs, start working transversus abdominis is going to switch off because it figures, "Something else is doing my job. I don't need to do it." and it switches off. So, we have to get this muscle working correctly and very specifically. We also need to work you in a neutral spine position. That basically means we don't want you in extension (arched back) because if you're in that extended position, that's putting more stress and strain on the spine. We don't want you in a flexed position (rounded back) because again, that's putting more stress and strain on your lower back as well. We want you in a neutral spine position, which is essentially the midpoint of the extremes of these two movements, as we found previously in Chapter 6. Neutral is where you feel the least amount of stress and strain through the spine. Once you find neutral, then we need to engage the core muscles in that neutral position.

The Best Core Exercise... Ever

There is a simple and effective exercise that most people can do to start engaging the core muscles more correctly. It's pelvic floor exercises AKA Kegels. As we learned earlier, the Transversus Abdominis and pelvic floor muscles work together as they are so internal. We can use the pelvic floor muscles to initiate a true core contraction.

This is a very different feeling to just pulling your stomach in, as it's very internal. But you are getting transversus abdominis switching on, however it takes some practice. For most people, these muscles are not doing what they need to do. You need to get them switched back on because your core should be on at a low level for you all day long. Transversus abdominis is an endurance muscle or a marathon muscle, it's not a sprint muscle. For example, think about working a fast twitch or sprint muscle like your biceps. If you were to do bicep curls, the muscle would switch on, switch off, switch on, switch off, as you raised your hand up and down. Transversus abdominis doesn't work like that. Transversus abdominis should be switched on just a little bit, so a low level of contraction, and then keep it on, on, on, on, on. It's more about endurance than speed.

Basically, because the transversus abdominis muscle is so internal, it works in conjunction with the pelvic floor muscles. I first teach these exercises lying down because there's no weight going through your body and particularly your spine, in a lying down position. The spine is also in a nice supported neutral posture position. Remember the position you started the knee rolling exercise in? That's how you're going to start with the core exercises too.

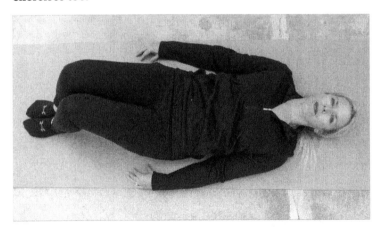

You're going to put your hands on your tummy. Put one hand on your tummy below your belly button and one hand on your tummy above your belly button. Don't push or press, you're just going to feel what the abdominal muscles are doing.

Now, try and suck in your lower tummy. It's like sucking in your gut. What happens with most people is that all the abs work together, because when your brain sends the message down to your stomach to say, "Okay, come on, switch on," all of the abdominals want to help. So, by consciously thinking about sucking your tummy in, you don't get a pure core contraction because everything works. The different visualization I give people is, "Okay, let's use a pelvic floor contraction." A nice way to do this is by using Kegels.

The pelvic floor muscles and this deep core muscle work together. We can do a pelvic floor contraction and get a sneaky switch on of transversus abdominis as well. Essentially, you're just going to imagine you're in the restroom, urinating, and stop the flow. That is what you're going to do to try to activate this muscle. Use the muscles that you'd use to stop peeing. Use those muscles to get a core contraction and start engaging transversus abdominis correctly. If you get the pelvic floor contraction, you will get a transversus abdominis contraction. It feels quite different to pulling your tummy in or sucking in the gut.

When I teach people this exercise, I say to them, "Okay, you're going to switch transversus on. Keep it switched on but keep breathing normally. You shouldn't be holding your breath because you can't walk around like that all day." You want to switch that muscle on and keep it on but keep breathing nice and normally. Hold the muscle contraction for about 10 seconds, then release it. Switch on again. Keep breathing normally. Hold for 10 seconds. Release it off. Try to do 10 repetitions at a time and try to do that every hour throughout the day. Yes, you need to be practicing it little and often. The key with transversus abdominis is it should be switched on for you all day long, and for most people, it's not because they're just not working it in the way that it's designed to be worked. Add in back pain, pregnancies or surgeries over the years, and transversus abdominis most likely started to switch off and off and off and off and off.

That's how you start to learn how to get the muscle switching on correctly. Have a practice now. You can check out a series of videos showing how you can start getting these muscles switched on in the book bonuses:

http://bit.ly/TE-bookbonuses

It is a good idea to get some guidance with regards to this if you are not sure if you are doing it correctly. You should not feel any pain or discomfort as you do any of these exercises. If you do, something's not right. You could be in a poor position or the muscles are not switching on correctly. If you're feeling discomfort, something is not okay, so certainly get that checked out with a physical therapist.

Why This Is Crucial For Your Recovery

Do I have to do these exercises for the rest of my life?

We all should be. It's when people don't do the things that they should, that they get pain and problems developing. If you have a dog or a cat, the first thing they do when they wake up is to stretch. No one has told them to, but they are innately designed to stretch and move their bodies. We should follow their lead and move our bodies as they were designed to move.

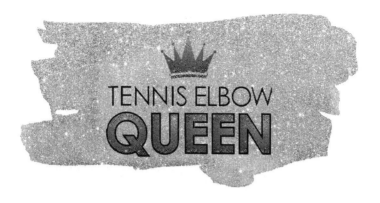

Success Story Snippet

66 My first session was wonderful, and Emma is great! Her approach is so different to every other therapist I've seen in the past. The last PT I saw made my pain much worse, after one session with Emma, I'm already feeling better! 99

– LP, male operating room nurse, 40s, USA

CHAPTER 9

Phase 4
Endurance And Function

One question I am asked all the time is, "Will it ever get better?" The simple answer is, yes, if you do the right things at the right time. This is then followed up with, "When will it get better?" And I would answer with, "Well, how long is a piece of string?" "How long is a piece of string?" they would repeat, "Well, I don't know, it depends." Exactly. That's my point. It depends on what you do, whether you do the right things, whether you do the wrong things. If you irritate it, it's going to take longer to get better than if you don't irritate it. Obvious really, right?

Generally, the length of time you have had tennis elbow symptoms before you start doing what I've recommended to you to do today is the length of time it's going to take for it to get better. So, if you've been suffering for 3 months, it can settle down in 3 months as long as you do the correct things. However, if you've had this for seven years, thankfully, it won't take seven years to settle down, and you will probably be better in around seven months. Now I know that still sounds a long time, but it's not seven years. Once we get up to the 12 month point and beyond, everyone can be better in 12 months, even if you've had it for three years, seven years or 20 years.

Most clients are better within six or seven months. Sometimes a little bit longer if it's a little more of a complex case. But some clients see a difference after just 1 session. Everybody is different and it just depends where you are on your journey. It depends what phase you are in.

How Long Does Each Phase Take?

This is another great question that I can also answer with "How long is a piece of string?" Everybody is different. Everybody's journey is slightly different but know that these are the phases that you have to go through. If you try and skip a phase, you're not going to heal. The symptoms will come back. You'll irritate it. These are the phases that you need to go through in this sequence in order to resolve tennis elbow, as though it was never there and return to doing everything you want to do without restrictions.

Some clients can get through Phase 1 and Phase 2 in two to three weeks and be pain free, have normal muscle tension and be ready for the strengthening phase. Other clients spend longer in phase one and two, particularly if they have been feeling the symptoms for a longer period of time, or have more structures involved, such as neck and shoulder as well as the elbow. This can also be the case with clients who experience nerve symptoms, as this can lengthen the time spent in phases one and two.

One of the original research articles that came out over 20 years ago, recommended that the most effective protocol for healing tendons was 12 weeks [35]. So, initially I taught my clients to do the strengthening exercises for three months, every single day, no days off, for three months. When they got through those three months, they'd be feeling fantastic by the end and then they would wean down.

Everybody is different. Some clients would say to me, I am never stopping these exercises because I feel good and I don't want the pain to ever come back. I'm going to keep doing it forever. Okay, fine. Keep going. If that works for you, brilliant. Some clients would say I'm going to do the exercises every other day, and that would keep them ticking over. Some clients would do them every week, once a week, just to keep topped up, others would be able to wean down completely and never have to do the exercises again.

Further research that came out more recently, purely about tendon healing, showed us that tendon healing takes a full year, that is, 12 months [36]. So, now I tell my clients to do the exercises every single day for a year. You're going to do them for a whole year because we know that by that point, your tendon pain is going to be completely resolved.

If the tendon is completely resolved, there is no chance of it coming back, and there's no reason why it should. Let's just say, for example, maybe you decide, "I'm going to take up tennis because my tennis elbow is all healed. I feel great. I am going to start playing tennis." And then you start feeling discomfort. Well, you know all the strategies to do straight away to nip it in the bud so that it does not come back because you know what to do.

Once you get established with the strengthening exercises, you will become pain free and that's when we start to think about getting you back to all the activities you want to do. To progress from Phase Three, strengthening, into Phase Four, building endurance and regaining function, you must have been completely pain free for a whole week doing all your normal activities. That means no twinge, no ache, no shadow of a something, no difference to the unaffected side at all. Once you reach that point, you are ready to regain your more intensive activities and we do this gradually and methodically, by only adding in one new exercise at a time for example, if you are returning to the gym or to weightlifting or gradually increasing the amount you play if you're returning to playing a musical instrument.

It's a slow and steady process to allow the tissue to accommodate to the new stresses and strains you are putting through them. I liken this process to that of a marathon runner. If you are brand new to marathon running, you don't get up one day and run 26.2 miles. You spend 6 months training and building up your stamina. You are essentially training the tissues of your body to tolerate the intensiveness of running 26 miles. We use this same principle to get you safely and comfortably back to your activities. It does require some patience, but we know that it takes 12 months for the tendon to fully resolve anyway, so what's the rush? Are you ready to begin your journey?

Nerve Mobilisations

This is the phase that I introduce specific nerve mobilizations, if not before. This tends to be a very individual issue and one that I currently guide clients through on a personal basis. The reason for this is that it is extremely easy to flare nerves up, by doing the wrong movement at the wrong time or even for the wrong amount of time. If you have nerve symptoms, get guidance from a specialist physical therapist on how best to settle your specific nerve issues.

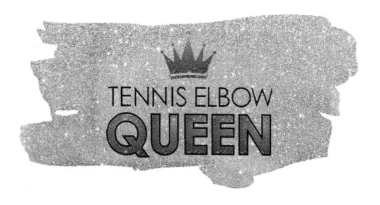

Success Story Snippet

66 Emma gets a gold star for giving me the right advice. The Dr was so impressed by how much my elbow had improved since my last appointment. I never thought I'd play hockey again, but I was back playing within 3 months of starting to work with Emma. I had no idea this would work from 5000 miles away. 99

– KH, female field hockey player, 40s, UK

CHAPTER 10

Next Steps

30-Day And 100-Day Guides

Next steps for you. You've got a lot of things that you can start today. Get going with the self-help strategies from Chapter 6, because every single one of those is helpful in its own way. If you only did one consistently, you would feel the benefit. Imagine if you do them all, how much better you are going to feel. The self-help strategies in Chapter 6 are going to get you through phase one. This is going to calm the symptoms down and it's going to allow you to start feeling a whole lot better.

First things first, start to implement everything I teach in this book. You'll find a handy 30-day plan at the back of this book. Once you've completed that, there's a 100-day Program to keep you going. This will give you guidance and structure to implement everything you've learned, without leaving anything out, so that you can start to feel better. Don't forget to grab the extra bonuses too:

http://bit.ly/TE-bookbonuses

Facebook Group

I would love it, if you haven't already, to come and join us on Facebook. I have a tennis elbow relief Facebook group. Buddy, my very first client, who you heard about earlier on, is in the group, and he is more than happy to talk to people about his experience resolving his elbow pain. The other clients who shared their success stories in this book, are in there too and want to give back.

Please use it, it's a great resource and starting point. It's free to join. I'm in there a lot of the time, so if you have a question, you can catch me there. I love answering questions. Questions are my favorite. So, please join my Facebook group so that you can be with other people who are in the same situation as you and other people who have been in the situation that you're in right now and they are through the other end. It's one thing to hear it from me, but another to hear it from them. They were in your shoes. They can tell you what it was like to go through it and to live it and to have it behind them. I invite you to join my Facebook group here:

https://www.facebook.com/groups/tenniselbowrelief

Helpful Hints Emails

I would really love for you to sign up for my helpful hints emails. You can do that in the Facebook group or by signing up for the book bonuses:

http://bit.ly/TE-bookbonuses

Tennis Elbow Relief Challenge

You can join the waiting list for the next Tennis Elbow Relief challenge inside the Facebook group. It's a three-day challenge. Basically, I teach you three different strategies. I get you to practice one per day with my guidance. Just doing one a day, so you can try it out, see if it works for you and add it in, then you can get a cumulative effect by the end of the week. There are always prizes for the challengers too. The Challenge Community Champion wins the heat pad that I recommend to my private clients and one lucky winner, who has participated in the challenge all week, wins a 30-minute consultation with me! You've got to be in it, to win it.

Website

Visit my website:

https://www.TennisElbowQueen.com

There you'll find a free eBook you can download and other helpful hints for home.

Online Tennis Elbow Relief Program

I have created an online Tennis Elbow Relief Program. This book has taken you through phase one, which is the most essential for beginning your healing journey. It sets your foundation. It gets you ready for the rest of the healing journey. It introduces you to several of the initial exercises in phase 2 and phase 3. Then you learn about how you progress through phase 4 to get back to doing all the things you want to be doing. I would love for you to come and join me in the comprehensive program that expands from this book. It works. It will take you through the whole journey with my guidance.

Learn more about the online Tennis Elbow Relief Program here:

http://bit.ly/TE-bookbonuses

Membership Group

There is an opportunity for you to join a small number of clients who are on their journey through my program, in a membership group. This group is much smaller than the Facebook group and members benefit from a weekly live call with me to answer all their questions. Email me if you are interested in this option and we can chat about your suitability for the group. Emma@ TennisElbowQueen.com

Your Opportunity To Work With Emma Beyond This Book

I really hope you've enjoyed reading this book as much as I have enjoyed writing it. You can probably tell I'm passionate about helping people. The reason I wrote this book was because I started to realize that I was saying the same things all the time to every single client, and I thought, I should write this down and get it out there, so that more people can be helped. So, here we are, this is how it was created. One-on-one consultations limit the number of people that I can help. In a platform like this I can help people all over the world, anytime of the day or night, the information is available.

However, there is more to come because there are more strategies that you need to do in Phase 2, like normalizing the soft tissues, phase three, strengthening, and then phase four, getting you back to everything you want to do. A lot of that information is going to come from the helpful hints emails. Please make sure that you sign up, so you don't miss out on any of that useful information. Remember I said if you miss strategies and try to jump ahead, you're just going to irritate your tendon and you're going to end up back in Phase 1. Let's not do that.

In the past I was very limited by seeing one-on-one clients.

There's only so much time in my day, especially when I'm helping my kids with online school at the moment. I work with a select number of clients, so if you absolutely want to work with me, one-on-one, there are possibilities for that. They are limited possibilities, but they are there if you need additional help. It may well just be a one-off consultation, just making sure that my program is right for your needs. Maybe you have something else going on or a different issue you want to ask me about. The option is there. Please email me to apply:

Emma@TennisElbowQueen.com

Don't forget, you can also get me in the Facebook group, so please join us. Don't let this be the end. What is it that Sir Winston Churchill said?

> 66 Now this is not the end.
> It is not even the beginning of the end.
> But it is, perhaps, the end of the beginning. 99

Everything you've just been through in this book will get you through Phase 1 and in to Phase 2. Let me take you through the complete Phase 2, Phase 3 and Phase 4. Let me get you to the point where tennis elbow is just a memory of the past, as it should be. Let's get you back to everything that you want to do as much as you want to do it. No restrictions. Don't live life in fear of pain. That's not living life. Let's not live life halfway, let's live life to the full. We're here for a very limited time. Let's enjoy it as much as we can.

Thank you so, so much for joining me in this book. I've absolutely loved taking you through the beginning of my program, as you can probably tell, this is what I love to do. If you have any comments, please feel free to share. I love questions, if I didn't explain something clearly enough, or if you need clarification on something or something could have been done in a better way, please don't hesitate to reach out because I'm really open to improving everything as much as possible. Please feel free to reach out, and I would absolutely love to see you in the program.

Telehealth

If you want to schedule a video consultation with me, feel free to email me. I can get your individual story. You can let me know what's going on. We can figure out the structure that's causing the issue and then make sure you're doing the right things to settle it down. So, feel free to reach out to me if you would like to schedule:

Emma@TennisElbowQueen.com

Thanks so much for reading. Take care and I hope to work with you soon.

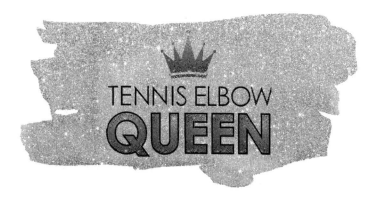

Success Story Snippet

❝I really enjoyed my sessions with Emma –
she is so patient and knowledgeable! I'm so glad
I found her – I had no idea that virtual sessions
could be so effective.❞

— AG, female housekeeper, 50s, USA

Success Stories

Buddy's Success Story

Hᴏ, I'ᴍ Bᴜᴅᴅʏ Gɪʙʙᴏɴs. I'm a professional drummer, and I can literally say that Emma Green saved my career. In 2008, I had drummed my right arm to death, and my elbow had completely quit working. It got to the point that I couldn't even lift a bottle of water with my right arm. It's not great for somebody in my line of work. After having gone to several surgeons, my wife and I went through everything we could do for my arm. We tried chiropractic, we tried doctors, we got cortisone shots, anything you can think of nearly. I found myself at an occupational therapist's office where Emma was working. Emma took an interest in my case. She realized that there was more going on than even the occupational therapists could figure out.

After having been told by all of these doctors that I probably only had about a 70% chance of recovery, Emma took me under her wing. She and I worked together for several months, to try to come up with a therapy that would work to solve my problem. I think the greatest thing about her was that she never stopped caring about actually healing my body. She took the time to literally create a brand-new technique, something that had never been done before on an elbow. She applied her knowledge of what works with the Achilles tendon to my elbow. I was not an easy patient for her because the things that she was doing didn't make a lot of sense to me, and I challenged her, shall we say, about why we were moving this way when I needed to move that way and things like that.

Ultimately, Emma basically got me to understand how the body worked together. During the course of our time together I went from being unable to pick up that bottle of water I mentioned, to what I consider completely healed. My elbow gives me zero trouble anymore. It's now been eleven years since I saw her professionally, and she is still someone that I consider a very dear friend. If you are looking for someone that will take a real interest in your case, whatever your case may be, Emma is the only one that I would ever refer you to. Ever. She is phenomenal. Thanks, Emma."

Sierra's Success Story

"Hi, my name is Sierra. I am one of the people that Emma helped get back onto the road to recovery. I came to Emma with tendonitis, tennis elbow, in my right forearm. I had had it for about three, maybe four years. It was very, very painful. I had sought care in other places, and while they had given me options for recovery, none of them worked.

I work in the entertainment industry. I work in costuming predominantly, but I also train stunts. One of the most important things is to have physical strength and for a particular stunt show I wanted to do, I needed to be able to do a pull up. Sadly, due to the tennis elbow, I couldn't make it through the audition.

I wish somebody had told me back when I first got injured, that you need to be looking for somebody who will both prioritize your recovery, as well as your success thereafter. That it's not just let's get you fixed, let's put a band aid on it and make it so that you can just function, but someone who will make sure that I can function, but then also thrive afterwards. That I can chase my goals, that I can be as athletic and as ambitious as I want to be. And that it's not just okay, now you can carry things. It's okay you can carry things, you can do pull-ups, you can do a stunt show, you can keep training, you can go back to kickboxing, like it doesn't matter.

If I could give advice to somebody starting out in seeking care, I would say, "Look for somebody who has a positive attitude for you." As I felt like I was often told I was too young to be injured. I shouldn't have a repetitive motion injury, and it made me feel like it was my fault when in reality yeah, I got hurt but I just needed someone to tell me how to get better. Fortunately, Emma was so kind and so capable of giving me both a roadmap to recovery, as well as the optimism I needed, which I believe further increased my healing.

If you're looking for treatment for a repetitive motion injury, or injury of any kind, I would say make sure not just where you want to return to, but where you want to go after that. Emma gave me the tools so that if it ever flares up again, or if I ever re-injure, I feel like I could help myself at least enough to get through or to regain some of the mobility that I may be losing."

Paul's Success Story

"Hi, MY NAME IS PAUL. I had tennis elbow for months, quite a bit of pain and getting nowhere. Healing was not happening. Then I was referred to Emma who immediately gave me a series of treatments that made all the difference. Emma is really knowledgeable, and she essentially cured me of my condition. I am back playing tennis, which for a while there I was wondering when and if that would ever happen. I was out for 11 months, and for six of those, I was with Emma and she got it done. Along the way, I also had some other muscle strains, hand and shoulder, hip flexor. She helped with all those. She's very knowledgeable. I could not recommend her more highly."

Will's Success Story

"As a very active person, contracting golfer's elbow was a huge hit to my ability to go about my usual day to day physical exercise & activities, which quickly took its toll on my mental health. I'm so grateful for having found Emma when I did, and enrolling on to her elbow programme; it quickly put my mind in a more positive space with the light at the end of the tunnel that I needed to focus on. After just a month on the course, I was mostly pain free day to day, and after 3 months I gradually started getting back to the things I love doing. I have every confidence that by following Emma's advice and programme, the months ahead will see me back to my prior levels of activity!"

Karen's Success Story

"My tennis elbow started in the summer of 2019 after doing too much gardening! I was struggling to pick up a glass of water and definitely couldn't lift anything heavier! I had no idea that virtual treatment could help. But, I had confidence in Emma and followed her instructions to the letter. Emma gets a gold star for giving me the right advice. The Dr was so impressed by how much my elbow had improved since my last appointment. I never thought I'd play hockey again, but I was back playing within 3 months of starting to work with Emma. I had no idea this would work from 5000 miles away."

Other Success Stories And Testimonials

Newly retired lady who loved playing golf developed tennis elbow in her non-dominant arm after increasing the number of days per week she was out on the golf course. After completing the Tennis Elbow Relief program, she was pain free and able to play golf as much as she wanted with no restrictions.

— JL

"She started going out with a friend a few weeks ago to practice softball. She said she is stretching, and her arm feels fine. Thank you so much for taking care of my daughter when everyone else said they couldn't! You are a miracle worker!"

— CC

"My first session was wonderful, and Emma is great! Her approach is so different to every other therapist I've seen in the past. The last PT I saw made my pain much worse, after one session with Emma, I'm already feeling better!"

— LP

Emma puts a lot of enjoyment into what she does — she listens, and it feels so good to finally be heard. It made me positive that I would heal — and I did."

— IC

"First I wanted to tell you that today's been a pretty good day so I've been really good about not being on the computer or texting on my phone hardly at all!! You are a wealth of information! I've NEVER heard such detailed info! Thank you again for always being available for questions, it means a lot!"

→ PT

"I like working with you – you are easy to deal with."

– NK

I really enjoyed my sessions with Emma – she is so patient and knowledgeable! I'm so glad I found her –
I had no idea that virtual sessions could be so effective."

– AG

"Virtual PT is way more convenient than I ever imagined. I don't have to travel anywhere."

– RC

"I have just told my Dr that I feel the best that I have ever felt – this is working! Awesome!"

– CH

Your 30-Day Starting Boost Plan
(Phase 1 And The Beginning Of Phases 2 And 3)

Y ou've learned a lot about tennis elbow and how to heal it. But what's next? You need to start implementing the self-help strategies I taught you in chapter 6.

But Emma, there are so, many of them, do I need to do all of them?

Do you want to heal your tennis elbow?

YES.

Every self- help strategy is in there for a reason. Start trying to skip, will lead to a longer healing time and potentially a worse outcome. Not good.

So, trust the process. This program has healed thousands of elbows. I've added, tweaked and evolved it over the years. Take the knowledge I've given you and heal this elbow. Don't hesitate to reach out if you need to. I can be reached here:

Emma@TennisElbowQueen.com

Add in the stretches you learned in Chapter 7. Build in the strengthening exercises from Chapter 8 and in the last chapter we touched on regaining endurance and function.

Before You Start

It's really important to understand why we are doing certain things, otherwise you may find yourself skipping over certain strategies after a few days, forgetting to do them after a while or never doing them from the start. If you find yourself wondering why you are doing a particular thing, head back to chapter 6 to refresh your memory as to why each section is needed.

The Basic Guidelines

These strategies need to be completed every single day with no days off. This is rehabilitation of your elbow. This is not fitness. We don't take rest days.

Try every single strategy. I've included everything I've ever used for every tennis elbow client I've helped. You may not need everything, but if you leave out something that you do need, you won't heal effectively. So, do it all to be on the safe side.

This book is not intended to diagnose any medical condition. See a doctor or other medical practitioner for that.

This book is not written for a specific person. I've included my vast knowledge of the many clients I have helped with their tennis elbows. I don't know you or your specific history. As such, you assume all risks associated with participating in a rehabilitation program, including getting clearance from your doctor prior to beginning any new exercise regime. You agree to hold harmless the author for any and all claims associated with participation in this rehabilitation program.

Worksheets

Fill out these charts to determine where you are starting from. Downloadable versions can be found at:

http://bit.ly/TE-bookbonuses

Weekly Planning

Scheduling your strategies into your day has proven to be a very effective way to be able to complete the program. See the daily checklist following and at:

http://bit.ly/TE-bookbonuses

HOMEWORK −
Last 7 Day Pain Episode Log Sheet for_____

Day	Severity of pain episode (1–10)	Time pain Occurred	Activity/What you were doing at the time to cause pain
Monday	i.e.7/10	8.30 am	Getting out of bed!
Tuesday			
Wednesday			
Thursday			
Friday			
Saturday			
Sunday			

Name: _____ Date: _____

PAIN DIAGRAM

On the diagrams below, mark where you are experiencing
pain, right now. Use the letters below to indicate
the type and location of your sensations.

Key: A – ACHE   **B** – BURNING   **N** – NUMBNESS
     P – PINS & NEEDLES   **S** – STABBING   **O** – OTHER

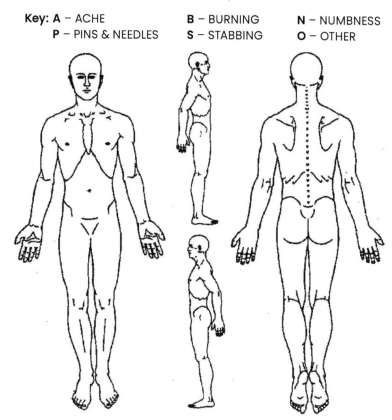

PAIN SCALE

Rate the severity of your pain by checking
one box on the following scale.

No Pain
                                                            Worst
                                                            Possible
                                                            Pain

0	1	2	3	4	5	6	7	8	9	10

Cardio Calendar

Here is my cardio calendar for you to use. You can download this at:

http://bit.ly/TE-bookbonuses

EMMA GREEN

TENNIS ELBOW QUEEN

Cardio Challenge

1	2	3	4	5	6	7
1 minute! Great start!	2 minutes! Keep it up!	3 minutes	4 minutes	5 minutes	6 minutes	7 minutes 1 week done!
8	**9**	**10**	**11**	**12**	**13**	**14**
8 minutes	9 minutes	10 minutes Double figures!	11 minutes	12 minutes	13 minutes	14 minutes 2 weeks!!
15	**16**	**17**	**18**	**19**	**20**	**21**
15 minutes Halfway there!	16 minutes	17 minutes	18 minutes	19 minutes	20 minutes	21 minutes 3 weeks!!!
22	**23**	**24**	**25**	**26**	**27**	**28**
22 minutes	23 minutes	24 minutes	25 minutes	26 minutes	27 minutes	28 minutes 4 weeks!!!!
29	**30**	**31**				
29 minutes Almost to your goal!!	30 minutes You did it!	30 minutes Whoop whoop!				

The Program

Follow this sample daily guideline for Phase 1 and Phase 2 self-help strategies. You can also download at:

http://bit.ly/TE-bookbonuses

Tennis Elbow Checklist - Phases 1 and 2 - Daily List

- **Heat** the elbow, neck, shoulder and forearm for 10 minutes, **at least** 5 times per day.

- **Neck Exercise** 10 times, at least 3 times per day.

- **Trigger point** the upper traps and forearm muscles after the heat.

- **Soft tissue massage** the forearm muscles after the heat.

- **Stretch** the upper traps, pecs, biceps, forearm, 30 second hold, at least 3 times per day.

- **Shoulder rolls** 10 reps at least 3 times per day.

- **Ice** the elbow for 3 days if you feel you have irritated it, then return to the heat.

- **Posture** Watch your posture, particularly when you are sitting. Set the timer on your phone for 20 minutes. When it goes off, stand up, sit down and resume a good posture.

- **Ergonomics** Use a wrist rest when you are typing and using the mouse.

- **Relative Rest** Avoid any activities that make it hurt.

- **Brace** Use a tennis elbow strap if you cannot avoid a painful activity. But only use it when you really need it as it will weaken the muscles.

- **Pills / potions / lotions** Take any pain medication, anti-inflammatories or muscle relaxers that have been prescribed to you by your doctor. If you try an over-the-counter medication, you should see a difference within 30 minutes - if not it's not helping maybe you don't need it.

- **Sleep** Get 8 hours per night.

- **Nutrition** Eat a healthy diet (eg Mediterranean) ensuring some protein at every meal and snack.

- **Hydration** 8 glasses of water per day.

- **Cardio** 30 minutes daily, ideally outside.

- **Progressive Relaxation** Every night before going to sleep.

- **Meditation** 15-20 minutes daily.

- **Visualization** Daily – start with a couple of minutes and build up. The more you do, the stronger the neural pathways stay.

Once you have decreased the muscle tension in the forearm, you are ready for Phase 3, strengthening. Remember, I mentioned this can take anywhere from a few days to a few months depending on the level of complexity of a case, how many different structures are affected and how long someone has suffered. Don't rush it. If you try to start the strengthening exercises too soon, you will flare it up. If that happens, you will then have to wait until it settles back down again which will take longer to ultimately heal.

If you are ready, let's move on.

The Next 100 Days Program

(Phase 3 And Phase 4)

This is where we start to add the strengthening exercises in. There is a very specific strengthening exercise to do that will heal the tendon. Follow this link to the video where I teach it:

http://bit.ly/TE-bookbonuses

Once you are doing the strengthening exercises, you will become pain free, if you haven't already. The strengthening exercise heals the tendon, and this is where the magic happens. You will need to slowly build up the weight as you get comfortable with the exercise and get stronger. Most clients who want to get back to low intensity activities will build up to using between 5- and 8-pound (2 to 3.5kg) dumbbells. Clients who want to return to mid-level intensity activities will build to between 8- and 12-pound (3.5 to 5.5kg) dumbbells. Clients who want to return to high intensity activities such as tennis or golf will build to between 12-to-15-pound (5.5 to 7kg) dumbbells.

Once you have been pain-free for a full week, doing all your normal daily activities, picking up your coffee cup or a bottle of water, lifting groceries or your laptop, turning a door handle or taking the lid off a jar, everything. Then, and only then, can you progress to Phase 4, regaining endurance, function and every-thing you want to be doing with no restrictions. This is again an incredibly strict timeline, as if you try to progress too soon, you will flare up again. That means that if you have gone for 6 days pain free but then feel a little discomfort on day 7, you have to start counting your week again. Don't try to rush this part, you've come so far, don't jeopardize your progress. Be truly honest with yourself.

Here's the checklist for Phases 1, 2 and 3. Download at:

http://bit.ly/TE-bookbonuses

Tennis Elbow Checklist - Phases 1, 2 and 3 - Daily List

- **Core exercises** try to switch on the core muscles 10 times every hour through the day. Hold each rep for 10 seconds, but don't hold your breath.

- **Heat** the elbow, neck, shoulder and forearm for 10 minutes, **at least** 5 times per day.

- **Neck Exercise** 10 times, at least 3 times per day.

- **Deep neck flexor exercises** do these, 10 reps 3 times per day, hold each rep for 10 seconds. Do them after the neck exercise.

- **Trigger point** the upper traps and forearm muscles after the heat.

- **Soft tissue massage** the forearm muscles after the heat.

- **Heavy Load Eccentrics** 3 sets of 15 twice a day, no days off.

- **Stretch** the upper traps, pecs, biceps, forearm (after each set of eccentrics), 30 second hold, at least 3 times per day.

- **Shoulder rolls** 10 reps at least 3 times per day.

- **Shoulder Blade exercises** aim for between 50 (lower intensity) and 100 (Higher intensity) reps per day, depending on what activities you want to get back to.

- **Rotator cuff rocks** aim for between 50 (lower intensity) and 100 (Higher intensity) reps per day, depending on what activities you want to get back to.

- **Ice** the elbow for 3 days if you feel you have irritated it, then return to the heat.

- **Posture** Watch your posture, particularly when you are sitting. Set the timer on your phone for 20 minutes. When it goes off, stand up, sit down and resume a good posture.

- **Ergonomics** Use a wrist rest when you are typing and using the mouse.

- **Relative Rest** Avoid any activities that make it hurt.

- **Brace** Use a tennis elbow strap if you cannot avoid a painful activity. But only use it when you really need it as it will weaken the muscles.

- **Pills / potions / lotions** Take any pain medication, anti-inflammatories or muscle relaxers that have been prescribed to you by your doctor. If you try an over-the-counter medication, you should see a difference within 30 minutes - if not it's not helping maybe you don't need it.

- **Sleep** Get 8 hours per night.

- **Nutrition** Eat a healthy diet (eg Mediterranean) ensuring some protein at every meal and snack.

- **Hydration** 8 glasses of water per day.

- **Cardio** 30 minutes daily, ideally outside.

- **Progressive Relaxation** Every night before going to sleep.

- **Meditation** 15-20 minutes daily.

- **Visualization** Daily - start with a couple of minutes and build up. The more you do, the stronger the neural pathways stay.

Bonus Section

Boost Your Immunity And Emma's Extra Energy

There's been no greater time where we all really need to boost our immunity, and these are really simple things that we can all do. Even if you just make one or two little changes, it's going to help. Please feel free to share it because it would be brilliant to get as many people as possible to boost their immunity.

I am going to share with you my eight tips for boosting your immunity and gaining extra energy.

Before lockdown, I was whizzing around getting kids to and from school, whizzing to and from work, whizzing everywhere. But I never felt like I had enough energy. I was always tired. It didn't matter what time I went to sleep. I would be dragging myself out of bed in the morning just so, so, tired. Going into lockdown, I thought, "Oh my goodness. How are we going to get through this?" But then within a few weeks of lockdown, I realized that I had so much more energy and felt so much better.

Our family relationships are better. I'm not screaming at the kids like I used to. Despite the fact that we've all been sitting on top of each other for the last 11 months now. The kids have not been physically in school and I've not been in the clinic. It was amazing. I started to think about what changes we had made, and I came up with this list of eight things that I want to share with you.

Daily Exercise

Let's go back to the olden days, pre-COVID. I thought I was pretty fit. I would exercise. I would always get at least 10,000 steps in every day. So, I thought I was in pretty good shape. But since going into lockdown, I now exercise at least once a day, maybe twice, maybe even three times per day. I used to think I couldn't fit it in. Daily exercise is one of the things that I think has really helped me.

Getting Into Nature

As you've learned, getting out into nature can be powerful. We are in lockdown. We're not going out and about like we used to, but we are walking the dog. When we walk the dog, we get out into nature. We see trees, flowers and other green things. It's really, really helpful for our mental health as well as our physical health to be outside and seeing green things. So, it's definitely something that I highly recommend. So, daily exercise, ideally outside, is an absolute must.

Daily Meditation

This is something that I kind of dabbled with in the past. I'd done it and I wasn't really very good at it because all these thoughts kept flying into my head, but I've really worked at it, and I completed a 21-day meditation challenge and I absolutely loved it. It only takes about 15 to 20 minutes and it's now part of my morning routine. I get up and do my exercise, then I will meditate for about 15 to 20 minutes. It's so immensely helpful just to get your head into the right place for the rest of the day.

Daily Journaling

Something else that also helps to set a positive focus for the day, is journaling. This is something that I started almost 2 years ago. I was going through quite a changing time in my life as I was leaving my hospital job after 25 years and going full-time into my own business. So, I journaled through that process and it was so helpful to get my thoughts down onto a piece of paper. It helps me immensely as I do have a gold, glittery notebook that I journal in with a matching gold pen. Just getting the thoughts out of your head and down on paper is really, really helpful.

Daily Multivitamins

I'd always given the kids supplements because my youngest is a bit of a picky eater, but when COVID hit, I started joining them and taking a daily multivitamin. We've also supplemented with chewable vitamin C as well. I take 350 milligrams of vitamin C in addition to the multivitamin. Vitamin C is a water-soluble vitamin so if you have too much of it, you essentially pee it out. Taking it has been helpful. The more I hear about supplements that can be helpful in the current situation, vitamin C is a big one. In addition to Vitamin D, get out in the sunshine if you can and zinc. Those three things seem to be pretty helpful right now with the current virus that's around. But obviously, always consult your doctor if you have questions.

Better Nutrition

Going back to before I left the hospital, I was going from the hospital to the clinic and then picking the kids up and then rushing around non-stop. Many times, in fact most workdays, I would not have lunch or if I did, it was on the run. I'd eat in the car or I'd eat while I was walking from the hospital to the clinic. So, it would just be something quick that I could grab. Not rubbish particularly, all the time, but just eating was an afterthought. It was like, "I've got to get from here to here. Let me go. What can I just snack on, on the way?" I hadn't realized how much it was draining my energy.

Since being in lockdown looking after the kids, they have to eat, or they turn into gremlins. If you've got kids, you know what I mean. We have to make sure we have 3 meals per day and we're having snacks too. A good breakfast in the morning and then I make sure they're having juices, fresh fruit, snacks and I'm there with them. So, actually just eating properly like I should do has been immensely helpful, but also eating more has given me more energy to be able to exercise.

Quarantini Time

This is something we've introduced obviously since being in quarantine. Quarantini time is essentially drinks at 6pm. Basically, what that means is the working day is done. Many times, in the past, the working day would spread out into however long I could make it. There were evenings that I would see clients at the clinic after 8pm or be writing notes or sending invoices well into the night. So, now, at six o'clock, the working day is done, the family comes together, and we have drinks at six.

Obviously, the kids are not drinking alcohol, and neither am I. In November 2019, I had a health scare and was admitted to the hospital for a suspected heart attack. Thankfully, I'm fine and the cause appeared to be burnout due to stress. For some reason, and it wasn't a volitional thing, like, "Oh, I'm not going to drink alcohol anymore because it's not good for me." I have completely gone off it. I can't even stomach the thought of drinking alcohol.

So, we've been trying out flavored sparkling waters, for

example a mandarin flavored sparkling water, or we've had grapefruit or blood orange, all of these really lovely flavors. But the important thing is the family comes together, even the dog, and we sit together outside and we talk about our day. It's just a really nice way for everyone to connect at the end of the workday. We're into rest and relaxation mode and just enjoying time together. I really view this time as precious time with my kiddos. They're off school, which was horrendous initially, but now it's let's just have fun together.

Gratitude

Finally, we are feeling grateful for what we have, and being able to spend this time together. For being healthy and keeping ourselves healthy. Gratitude plays a big part.

I really hope these tips help you. I do have so much more energy now. I realized the other day, I barely yawn. I'm not really tired and I sleep really well. I'm up way before six every morning to get up and out to do my exercise and I'm not dragging myself out of bed. Most days I'm awake before my alarm and then I'm just up and ready for the day. I hope that you can join me in feeling this amount of energy and feeling so great. If you have any questions, please don't hesitate to reach out.

FAQs

How does your Program help tennis elbow?

The Tennis Elbow Relief Program is an all-encompassing, hurt to healed system that was developed in response to a need for a better way to treat and heal tennis elbow. It was extensively researched and is evidenced based. It continues to evolve and change as new research comes out, or more effective techniques are developed. This will never stop. It is a comprehensive treatment program that anyone can follow and find success with.

What makes your Program different to other treatments out there?

My Program addresses the nervous system, where most other treatments don't. I also created and developed a logical system of treatment which is segmented into Phases. Each phase builds on the healing of the previous phase to solidify your progress. If you commit to the process, this is a no-fail system. You just have to follow the Program.

Questions to ask your healthcare provider

- How many tennis elbow clients do you see each week?
- What exercises will you start me with?
- How will you address the nerve symptoms?
- How long will I need to do the exercises for?

You want to work with someone who treats multiple tennis elbow clients each week, that is someone who recognizes the involvement of the spine. Someone who will give you advice regarding settling the nervous system down and who is aware of the research proving that tendons take 12 months to fully resolve. If you get these answers to these questions, jump right into their care. If you don't hear these answers, they may not be the specialist you are searching for and will be unable to give you the specialist knowledge and treatment that you require to fully resolve.

Do you suggest doing stretches in the morning even when you don't have any pain?

Yes, absolutely. What a great question. There are two different sets of exercises that I do every morning and evening. They are really good for spine health. If you start doing things now that are good for your spine health, in 20, 30, 40 years' time, your spine is going to be thanking you for sure. One of them is the knee rolling from side to side that ensures you're getting a good range of motion through the lower back joints, and it keeps the joints healthy. 10 in the morning, 10 at night. It'll take you 10 seconds each time. It's super fast. The other is the neck exercise.

Should we stretch before or after exercise?

The answer is both, but in different ways.

An athlete knows that it's important to warm up tissues before exercising maximally. You will not see an elite sprinter go from the team bus to their 100m race on the track without spending a considerable amount of time preparing both mind and body. But how much stretching should we be doing before exercise?

The current consensus is that we should prepare the body

specifically for the type of activity we are about to do using a dynamic warm up of stretches and movements that mimic the movements we will be doing. So, a warmup for a golfer would be very different to the warmup for a runner.

Elite athletes then use a cool down to prevent lactic acid build up. Their cool down will include a period of time performing gentle cardio, followed by a prolonged stretch session. This is when they would tend to use more static stretches as they work on flexibility.

My program advocates stretches after strengthening exercises to ensure that we reduce the muscle tension back down after increasing it with the strengthening motions.

Does my insurance cover me coming to see you?

When I hear these words, I always ask "Is whether or not a therapist takes your insurance, the most important factor in deciding to work with someone?"

I'll give you an example from my own life.

My son needed to see a doctor and after thoroughly researching the best doctor in this particular specialty in our area, I found the doctor that I wanted to help my son. He had great reviews from other parents, but was completely out of network, or cash-based. In other words, visits to see him would not be covered by our health insurance. So, what did I do? Start my search over and settle for an in-network doctor, just so that I could use our insurance? Heck, no. I wanted my son to see the best doctor he could. Someone who could help him. I wasn't going to let my insurance company dictate the quality of care that my son would receive. No way.

There's a saying "You get what you pay for." This doesn't

just apply to products like shoes and burgers but applies just as much to services like the guy you hire to paint your house or your healthcare provider. Whether you drive through the Golden Arches or head to a celebrity chef's newest gourmet restaurant, you know there will be a difference in the cost of your burger and that will be reflected in the quality of the food and the overall experience. Or how about the last time you shopped for a new phone, does anyone choose a flip phone over a shiny, new smart phone? None of us wants to have to take the cheaper option. But that doesn't mean we don't want value; we most certainly do.

If you have been to a physical therapy clinic in the past, think back to that experience. Was it a "Mill-like" clinic with cookie cutter care? How much time did you actually get to spend one to one with the qualified clinician? Not much? The reason is that in order to keep their doors open these In-Network clinics have to cram patients in and limit the dedicated one to one time with the clinician. One of my In-Network clinic owner friends just sent me a photo of a check they just received from an insurance company, who shall remain nameless, for the princely sum of $0.01. One penny. That's how much they valued the hard work, dedication and 7 years of education leading to a doctorate degree, that my friend was providing to their members. Could anyone live off a check for $0.01? It's no wonder more and more providers are having to switch to being out of network or cash based.

What about patients though? I know a gentleman who has a deductible of $15,000. $15k. That means that he has to pay the first $15,000 of his healthcare cost before his health insurance kicks in. A lady I know has a $75 copay for physical therapy. Another clinic friend of mine has a patient who has a

$150 copay. That means they pay $150 each time they go to see the In-Network clinic to receive the cookie cutter care. Do you think they're going to get back to doing everything they want to achieve before the 12 sessions of physical therapy that their insurance company begrudgingly allows them each year runs out? Not even close.

Many people are switching to Health Maintenance Organizations (HMOs) as a way to lower their monthly premiums but are then choosing to pay cash for specialist services that their HMO doesn't provide.

I wouldn't compromise the healthcare of my son, why do people compromise their own care?

I can get Physical Therapy much more cheaply. What makes you different?

Not all Practitioners are created equally. In-Network therapists are limited in the scope of practice they can utilize. They may even be limited in the body part that can be treated. For example, someone may be suffering with right elbow pain, so the doctor orders Physical Therapy for the right elbow pain. The In-Network therapist has no choice but to treat the right elbow as that is what the doctor ordered and if the insurance company sees any other body part treated in notes, they will refuse to make payment, leading to the patient being responsible for the cost of the session anyway. But what if the right elbow pain is due in part to a problem in the neck? The right elbow can be worked on as long as you like, but if that's not the cause of the issue, it'll never get better, no matter how many sessions you try. It would be far more advantageous to get a fully comprehensive evaluation from the start, and to determine the root cause of the problem. Then the appropriate plan can be devised to fully and completely alleviate the issue and rehabilitate the tissue to allow full recovery and return to all goals, without fear of the problem recurring.

I was asked this question recently by a private client and I gave him the above answer. This wasn't satisfactory to him. He made me think much more deeply about what actually makes me different. This is when I realized that what makes me different, is the fact that I address the nervous system from day 1! Most general healthcare providers don't address the nervous system AT ALL, let alone from day 1 and throughout their entire plan of care.

Can Foam Rolling help?

Some people swear by foam rolling, other people hate it. My view is, try it and see. I actually sometimes recommend people try the rolling pin out of their kitchen. Bruising is a sign of tissue damage, so that wouldn't be good, but other than that, if it feels good to you, no problem, use it. If you've tried it and you don't like it, don't worry, it's just not the best treatment technique for you, but there are plenty of others to choose from.

Does Kinesio Tape work for tennis elbow?

Kinesio tape, KT tape, Rock Tape these are all brand names of similar products. Kinesio tape was the original and first, so I will use that name for this section. When Kinesio Tape first came out, I was skeptical about it and especially with some of the claims that they were making with it. At the time, I was working with a guy who had had a knee surgery, and he had the most swollen knee that I'd ever seen. He was really, really struggling.

One of the claims Kinesio Tape makes, is that it takes down

swelling. This is due to the way the glue is applied in a wave formation on the back of the tape. This lifts up the layers of tissue to allow free flow of fluid underneath. As I had tried many different strategies with this guy's knee, to no avail, I said, "This is supposed to reduce swelling. I don't know whether it works, but let's try it." I put the Kinesio Tape on to reduce the swelling in his knee, and he came back the next week, and we were both amazed at his improvement because the swelling had gone down significantly. It does work to reduce swelling.

The other really big success I had with Kinesio Tape was with a lady who had rib pain. She had had a surgery and she was getting unremitting nerve pain around her ribs. Her surgeon had told her they thought the nerves had been caught in the scar, and there was nothing they could do. She had to live with it. It's one of those things. She'd had this pain for 18 months. She came to see me for something completely unrelated, I was using Kinesio Tape on her leg for a different issue, and she told me about her rib pain. I thought about it and we decided to give it a try. I put it on her ribs, tensioned it in a particular way that I thought would take the tension off her nerves. When I had placed the tape, she just looked at me, and said, "I have no pain. My pain is gone." She cried. I cried. It was amazing. Since then, I do actually call it magic tape.

Having said all of this, I have unfortunately found minimal benefit for tennis elbow sufferers with the use of Kinesio tape. Although, if you have used it and found it beneficial, I would say keep using it.

What is the recommended usage?

I would say when you need it. Try and not use it all the time. If you're using it all the time, the skin is going to break down, and then you won't be able to use it. That can be a problem. You don't want to get skin breakdown. That's the biggest concern with using any kind of tape because if your skin breaks down, you're going to have to stop using it. You would also not be able to use heat or ice until the skin healed. After you've taken the tape off, just do a little rub through with milk of magnesia. That really helps the skin.

If you know you're going to be doing something where you're going to be uncomfortable, put it on, but ideally, we want to get you to the point where you don't have to use it. There's clearly something that's irritated. There's something that's unhappy. So, let's figure out what that is and how to fix it, and then you won't need to use the tape anymore.

Should I do yoga?

Yoga is wonderful but there are many forms of yoga and not every one of them may be right for you. A gentle class specific for beginners would be the best place to start your practice if you are brand new to this form of exercise. There are even chair yoga classes, which make yoga accessible to many people.

Some people with tennis elbow are able to continue a modified yoga practice, whereas others find it irritating to their elbow and have to stop. My advice would be to try it and see. Listen to your body. We should all listen to our bodies much more than we do. They give us lots of really good information, but we're not always listening or wanting to hear what they are telling us. We perhaps need to pay a little more attention to what's going on inside. Our bodies are great healers, as long as we give them what they need.

References

1. Calfee, RP, Patel, A, DaSilva, MF, Akelman, E Management of lateral epicondylitis: current concepts *J. Am. Acad. Orthop. Surg.*2008 1619–29

2. Cutts, S, Gangoo, S, Modi, N, Pasapula, C Tennis elbow: A Clinical review article *J. Orthop.* 2019 203–7

3. Kongsgaard M, Kovanen V, Aagaard P, et al.Corticosteroid injections, eccentric decline squat training and heavy slow resistance training in patellar tendinopathy. *Scand J Med Sci Sports.* 2009 790–802

4. Nichols AW. Complications associated with the use of corticosteroids in the treatment of athletic injuries. *Clin J Sport Med.* 2005;15(5):370–375

5. Brinks A, Koes BW, Volkers ACW, Verhaar JAN, Bierma-Zeinstra SMA Adverse effects of extra-articular cosrticosteroid injections: a systematic review. *BMC Musculoskelet Disord.* 2010 206

6. Coombes BK, Bisset L, Brooks P, Khan A, Vicenzino B. Effect of corticosteroid injection, physiotherapy, or both on clinical outcomes in patients with unilateral lateral epicondylalgia: a randomized controlled trial. *JAMA.* 2013 461–9

7. Connell D, Burke F, Coombes P et-al. Sonographic examination of lateral epicondylitis. *AJR Am J Roentgenol.* 2001 777–82

8. Martel MO, Finan PH, Dolman AJ, Sudramanian S, Edwards RR, Wasan AD, Jamison RN Self-reports of medication side effects and pain-related activity interference in patients with chronic pain: A longitudinal cohort study. *Pain.* 2015 1092–1110

9. Maffulli N, Moller HD, Evans CH Tendon healing: can it be optimised? *British Journal of Sports Medicine* 2002 315–316

10. Sharma P, Maffulli, N Biology of tendon injury: Healing, modeling and remodeling *Journal of musculoskeletal & neuronal interactions* 2005 181–90

11. Chanda ML, Alvin MD, Schnitzer TJ, Apkarian AV Pain characteristic differences between subacute and chronic back pain *J Pain* 2011 792–800

12. Öhberg L, Lorentzon R, Alfredson H Eccentric training in patients with chronic Achilles tendinosis: normalised tendon structure and decreased thickness at follow up *British Journal of Sports Medicine* 2004 8–11

13. Walz DM, Newman JS, Konin GP, Ross G Epicondylitis: Pathogenesis, Imaging, and Treatment *RadioGraphics* 2010 167–184

14. Booth PW Physiological and biochemical effects of immobilization on muscle. *Clinical Orthopedics and Related Research* 1987 15–20

15. Lindboe CP, Platou CS Effects of immobilization of short duration on muscle fibre size. *Clinical Physiology* 1984 183

16. Miles MP, Clarkson PM, Bean M, Ambach K, Mulroy J, Vincent K Muscle function at the wrist following 9 d of immobilization and suspension. *Med Sci Sports Exerc.* 1994 615–23

17. Clark BC, Manini TM, Hoffman RL, Russ DW Restoration of voluntary muscle strength after 3 weeks of cast immobilization is suppressed in women compared with men. *Arch Phys Med Rehabil.* 2009 178–80

18. Dingemanse R, Randsdorp M, Koes BW, Huisstede BM Evidence for the effectiveness of electrophysical modalities for treatment of medial and lateral epicondylitis: a systematic review. *Br J Sports Med.* 2014 957–65

19. Bisset L, Paungmali A, Vicenzino B, Beller E A systematic review and meta-analysis of clinical trials on physical interventions for lateral epicondylalgia. *Br J Sports Med.* 2005 411–22

20. Lai WC, Erickson BJ, Mlynarek RA, Wang D Chronic lateral epicondylitis: challenges and solutions. *Open Access J Sports Med.* 2018 243–251

21. Titchener AG, Fakis A, Tambe AA, Smith C, Hubbard RB, Clark DI Risk factors in lateral epicondylitis (tennis elbow): a case-control study. *Journal of Hand Therapy* 2012 159–64

22. Kim GK The Risk of Fluoroquinolone-induced Tendinopathy and Tendon Rupture: What Does The Clinician Need To Know? *J Clin Aesthet Dermatol.* 2010 49–54.

23. Järvinen TA Neovascularisation in tendinopathy: from eradication to stabilisation? *British Journal of Sports Medicine* 2020 1–2

24. Grigg NL, Wearing SC, Smeathers JE Eccentric calf muscle exercise produces a greater acute reduction in Achilles tendon thickness than concentric exercise *British Journal of Sports Medicine* 2009 280–283

25. Yang S, Chang MC. Chronic Pain: Structural and Functional Changes in Brain Structures and Associated Negative Affective States. *Int J Mol Sci.* 2019 3130

26. Woolf CJ. Central sensitization: Implications for the diagnosis and treatment of pain. *Pain.* 2010;152(2 Suppl) S2–15

27. Gunn CC, Milbrandt WE. Tennis elbow and the cervical spine *Can Med Assoc J.* 1976 803–809

28. Smeets JS, Horstman AM, Vles GF, Emans PJ, Goessens JP, Gijsen AP, van Kranenburg JM, van Loon LJ Protein synthesis rates of muscle, tendon, ligament, cartilage, and bone tissue in vivo in humans *PLoS ONE* 2019 14

29. Seminowicz DA, Wideman TH, Naso L, Hatami-Khoroushahi Z, Fallatah S, Ware MA, Jarzem P, Bushnell MC, Shir Y, Ouellet JA, Stone LS Effective Treatment of Chronic Low Back Pain in Humans Reverses Abnormal Brain Anatomy and Function *Journal of Neuroscience* 2011 7540–7550

30. Young SN, Biologic effects of mindfulness meditation: growing insights into neurobiologic aspects of the prevention of depression *J Psychiatry Neurosci.* 2011 75–77

31. Ranganathan VK, Siemionow V, Liu JZ, Sahgal V, Yue GH From mental power to muscle power--gaining strength by using the mind. *Neuropsychologia.* 2004 944–56

32. Ayala Fde Baranda Andujar PS Effect of 3 different active stretch durations on hip flexion range of motion. *J Strength Cond Res.* 2010 430–436

33. Hodges PW, Richardson CA Inefficient muscular stabilization of the lumbar spine associated with low back pain A motor control evaluation of transversus abdominis. *Spine* 1996 2640–2650

34. Hides J, Richardson C, Jull G Multifidus muscle recovery is not automatic after resolution of acute, first-episode low back pain *Spine* 1996 2763–9

35. Alfredson H, Pietila T, Jonsson P.*et al* Heavy-load eccentric calf muscle training for the treatment of chronic Achilles tendinosis *Am J Sports Med* 1998 360–366

36. Sharma P, Maffulli N Tendon Injury and Tendinopathy: Healing and Repair *The Journal of Bone and Joint Surgery* American volume 2005 187–202

37. Garg R, Adamson G, Dawson P, Shankwiler J, Pink M. A prospective randomized study comparing a forearm strap brace versus a wrist splint for the treatment of lateral epicondylitis. *Journal of Shoulder and Elbow Surgery* 2010 508–12

Acknowledgments

**This book would not be in your hands
but for the following people:**

- My family for bearing with me whilst I wrote my book. I know it was tough at times, boys, but we made it through.

- Buddy Gibbons, the inspiration for finding the solution to tennis elbow and going along with my different ideas until we got it right!

- Dr Annette Billings for entrusting me with her wonderful clients and her deep friendship. It means more to me than you know.

- Leesa Ellis, my book mentor, for holding my hand through the process of writing my first book. I could not have done this without your guidance!

- Kris Rennig for making sense of my writing and editing out a million "so's" and exclamation points!!!!!!!

- Paul Gough, my business coach, who lit the spark under my arse to actually write this book.

- Dean Volk for his constant prodding to get the writing done.

- John Takemura for taking a chance on a crazy English physio and putting her in an office with Jackie Chipot!

- Beth Moser Chang for the amazing photos, thank you friend. Your work astounds me every time.

- Sam Griffiths for the wonderful illustrations and my Tennis Elbow Queen logo. You truly are Miss Chief Creative.

- "Sir" Stephen Bridgeman for making me the Queen, twenty years after you made me a Spice Girl. You really really know how to make a girl happy!

About The Author

Emma found physical therapy through being a patient herself at age 13 – after the doctor told her that she needed to give up gymnastics – which she thankfully didn't have to do! She quickly realized that physical therapy was the career for her as she thoroughly enjoys helping people and solving health and wellness challenges, many times surprising the medical doctors by how well her clients recover! A common phrase you'll hear her say is "I love proving the doctors wrong!" when clients are told they will have to give up something they love, like playing a musical instrument, going to the gym or even working on a computer!

Emma gets it. She has faced many of the same challenges you face today. She knows what it's like to be scared about whether you'll ever be able to be active again. It's physically and emotionally devastating to not be able to participate in the activities you love. Let's be honest - it's scary when you don't know how you're ever going to get back to doing the things you

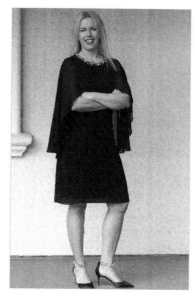

long to do, especially if your doctor only offered pain medications or injections and you're so busy with work and family that it's hard to find time to search for other solutions. Emma has figured out how to keep her clients doing the things they love and being active for life. That's why she created her Tennis Elbow Relief Program - to make sure that no one has to suffer from a lack of care or being told they have to stop doing what they love, like she did as a 13-year-old.

If you're serious about getting back to the activities you love, then Emma Green is the guide for you.

Emma graduated from Manchester University, England as a Physical Therapist and gained a Masters degree in Sports Medicine. She is now dual qualified being both a licensed Physical Therapist (USA) and a Physiotherapist (UK) along with being certified in Clinical Pilates through the Australian Physiotherapy and Pilates Institute.

Emma's early career saw her traveling worldwide with numerous national sports teams, the highlight of which was working at the London 2012 Olympic Games. She now lives with her family in Southern California.

Find her at:
https://www.TennisElbowQueen.com

Facebook:
https://www.facebook.com/EmmaGreenOnline

Instagram:
https://www.instagram.com/emmagreenonline

Printed in Great Britain
by Amazon

47629653R00115